You Can Be as Young as You Think

Prentice Hall LIFE

If life is what you make it, then making it better starts here.

What we learn today can change our lives tomorrow. It can change our goals or change our minds; open up new opportunities or simply inspire us to make a difference. That's why we have created a new breed of books that do more to help you make more of *your* life.

Whether you want more confidence or less stress, a new skill or a different perspective, we've designed *Prentice Hall Life* books to help you to make a change for the better. Together with our authors we share a commitment to bring you the brightest ideas and best ways to manage your life, work and wealth.

In these pages we hope you'll find the ideas you need for the life *you* want. Go on, help yourself.

It's what you make it

* * *

You Can Be as Young as You Think

Six Steps to staying younger and feeling sharper

Tim Drake and Chris Middleton

PEARSON
Prentice Hall
LIFE

Harlow, England • London • New York • Boston • San Francisco • Toronto • Sydney • Singapore • Hong Kong
Tokyo • Seoul • Taipei • New Delhi • Cape Town • Madrid • Mexico City • Amsterdam • Munich • Paris • Milan

PEARSON EDUCATION LIMITED

Edinburgh Gate
Harlow CM20 2JE
Tel: +44 (0)1279 623623
Fax: +44 (0)1279 431059
Website: www.pearsoned.co.uk

First published in Great Britain in 2009

© Pearson Education Limited 2009

The right of Tim Drake and Chris Middleton to be identified as authors of this work has been asserted by them in accordance with the Copyright, Designs and Patents Act 1988.

ISBN: 978-0-273-72270-0

British Library Cataloguing-in-Publication Data
A catalogue record for this book is available from the British Library

Library of Congress Cataloging-in-Publication Data
A catalog record for this book is available from the Library of Congress

10 9 8 7 6 5 4 3 2 1
13 12 11 10 09

Typeset in 10pt IowanOldStyle by 3
Printed by Ashford Colour Press Ltd., Gosport

The publisher's policy is to use paper manufactured from sustainable forests.

'Every child is born an artist.
The trick is to remain an artist.'
Pablo Picasso

'Youth is a wonderful thing. What a crime to waste
it on children'.
George Bernard Shaw

To my family, the incomparable Lizzie, and the egregious Tansy and Lettice.

And in loving memory of Chris Gates, who died a boy, aged 57. **Tim Drake**

To my wonderful wife, Valerie, and my lovely children, Jeremy and Antony. **Chris Middleton**

Contents

Acknowledgements

We have been helped in writing our book by a number of Young Brained enthusiasts. Thanks go first and foremost to our publisher and the early belief shown by Rachael Stock in our project. Her guiding hand and sure touch have been essential to the book you have in your grasp today. Our literary agent, Adrian Weston of Raft has encouraged us all the way. If there were prizes given out for youthful enthsiasm, Adrian would be at the top of the podium.

This book benefits enormously by being able to quote from exclusive socio-cultural data which is not normally available for publication.

We would like, therefore, to raise our hats high to Patrick Degrave in his capacity as Chairman of the Management Board of Sociovision – the acclaimed international socio-cultural research institute.

Several people read drafts of the book and contributed wise words when they were most needed. Juergen Schwoerer is a very good friend and originator of the 'YQ' concept. We valued his every word. Thanks in particular to Tansy, a Young Birthdayed Young Brain who read some early drafts and made helpful suggestions. And to Lizzie, a more mature Young Brain, for her insightful input.

As always, book writing takes enormous patience and endurance. Not, we hasten to add, for the authors. We had the easy, fun part. No, it's our respective families who've had to suffer the long hours and missed opportunities.

So thanks to Valerie, Jeremy and Antony, and to Lizzie, Tansy and Lettice.

It's great being back with you.

Tim and Chris

Introduction

This book is about your youth. It's about your desire to hold on to it and avoid the painful process of ageing. At the same time, it's also about being sharper and happier as you mature.

You Can Be as Young as You Think carries an uplifting, yet simple, message. Ageing is in the mind. If you think youthful thoughts you can remain young – and rejuvenate. Think younger and you will be more alert mentally. More importantly, you will genuinely act younger. By both thinking and acting younger, you will lead a wiser, more rewarding and fulfilled life.

You may feel that your youth is starting to seep away. And maybe you feel that life once seemed much simpler. The reality is that life *was* much simpler – because, when you were younger, you were *better at living it*. Somewhere along the line you lost the ability to think and act as youthfully as you once did. You lost the Wisdom of Youth.

This is a big story. It blows wide open many of our assumptions about ageing. Contrary to popular belief:

- Ageing is more about how you think than how you look.

- How you think is not determined by the inexorable march of time: at any given age, you can choose to think 'young' (as a Young Brain) or you can choose to think 'old' (as an Old Brain).

- Most of the time, people don't choose to think old thoughts, this happens by default. Remarkably, this inadvertent mental ageing process can start as young as 20!

- Wisdom is not only about the experience you accumulate as you age. You were born with natural wisdom – the wisdom of youth – which can be lost as you age.

● For many of us, the wisdom gained as we mature does not offset the loss of the Wisdom of Youth. The result is that, over time, we get Old Brained; we get worse at living our lives.

The Old Brained mindset of people who have lost the natural Wisdom of Youth holds very real perils; it is plagued by regrets for lost youth, by the fear of getting old and by the anxiety of being left behind by a changing world. Old Brained people are characterised by grumpiness, introspection and narrow-mindedness. They tend to be backward-looking; they lack creativity, humour and, above all, joy.

This book's aim is to steer you away from these perilous geriatric waters. Instead, we want to stimulate you to take the actions necessary to develop a Young Brain – full of imagination, spark, friendship and pleasure.

To support our message, we'll be showing you robust research figures throughout the book, which clearly show that people's attitudes and approach to life start to get more Old Brained quite early on in their lives. For some it starts as early as 18, for others 25 and others later still.

Meanwhile, a lucky few never seem to lose the Wisdom of Youth. Our objective is to help you join their ranks by enabling you to rediscover the Wisdom of Youth. By adopting young attitudes and approaches to life you can avoid a prematurely ageing brain. And stay Young Brained for ever.

Yes, the good news is that it is possible to regain what you thought you'd lost for ever. You can reject the deterministic downward spiral of ageing. You can become youthful again by deliberately choosing to have a Young Brain. We will show you Six Steps – the six wisdoms of youth – to achieve this.

The news gets even better. The Six Steps we describe in this book are open to anyone. It is possible for everyone – whatever their age and starting point – to think young, to revitalise and rejuvenate their lives. And, what is more, retaining or regaining your youth requires minimal financial resources. Take the time to work through this book and we will hand you the blueprint for success.

If you have picked up this book, it's probably because you realise that you are not where you want to be – or, at the very least, are worried about where you are heading. Possibly you feel old before your time, somehow less alert and fresh. Or slightly envious of people around you whose very personalities are somehow more youthful and vibrant. Something needs changing.

Of course, change is never easy and we are not promising that you'll become younger and feel sharper overnight. However, by understanding and injecting the six wisdoms of youth into your daily life, you will slowly rediscover freedom – the freedom to be open, flexible and exuberant. You will have the strategies at hand to tap into youthful energy and enjoy new access to the world and the people around you. In short, *You Can Be as Young as You Think* will give you the possibility to live life to the full and leave a lasting legacy.

This book is also about helping you to regain your youth by getting you to make the right choices. You can *choose* to remain relevant or you can decide to slip slowly into passivity and irrelevance. You can *choose* between making friends with new and interesting people or hanging on to a handful of cronies in your close social circle. It's *up to you* to either enhance your mental approach to life in order to live everything the 21st century has to offer – or retreat into the backwaters of fearful and stagnant thinking.

Finally, we lay down a challenge: are you satisfied that you are doing everything possible to be the best you can be? If not, read on and change your life for ever!

How to use this book

This book challenges you to change your thinking at a profound level. And in doing so to become younger, wiser and happier. But we realise we are asking a lot of you. It requires real courage to remould your thoughts and actions and there are lots of barriers that will get in your way. You'll not be surprised to learn, therefore, that to achieve rejuvenation requires you to commit both time and effort to the journey. You will have to be ready to look closely at your self-image and be prepared to do some internal work. You will need to alter how you think about yourself and the world around you. Also you'll have to reinforce all of this by changing some age-old behaviours. Once again, we know that this will require courage – and wisdom. We understand this because we face the same challenges as you.

Stripped back to its basics, this book has only two elements:

1 An explanation of how and why a new mental approach can make you younger. (Here we give you the rationale for change and the motivation to make it happen.)

2 Practical steps to change your mindset – injections of youthful wisdom. (Here we give you a realistic roadmap to transform your life.)

As you read on, we want you to get involved with this material, interact with it and own it. The easiest way to do this is to make this book your own. For once, forget about passing it on to someone else. This book is for you to personalise. So get out your pens and highlighters, and really go to work on the content. Make notes to yourself in the margin, underline, circle – whatever. Just make sure that you really feel you are doing this for yourself ... and for your future, younger self.

Much of what you'll be challenged to do will be away from this book, in your everyday life. Injecting the Wisdom of Youth means rising to challenges and meeting goals. For each Wisdom of Youth, we invite you to answer 'Challenges' and go out there and take actions: learning by doing.

So you are holding both an inspirational book and a workbook. Use it as a jumping-off point and also a guide to come back to when doubts set in.

We all like shortcuts, but remember that the amount of rejuvenation and revitalisation you gain will depend on just how much you are willing to participate in, and persist with, the actions we suggest.

It's important to understand that each of the wisdoms of youth are related, but not prioritised. Only you can decide what you need to do, based on your own personal situation. You can tackle the wisdoms of youth all at once or one by one. However, our suggestion would be to read all six strategies, identify a couple where you feel you have most to gain, and focus on those two for the next few months. Then, once these two are well embedded, go on to others.

There are no quick fixes and no instant youth. But if you want to avoid the negatives of ageing, you can give yourself a winning chance. Armed with this book and with new conviction and courage, you can rejuvenate your whole approach to, and enjoyment of, life. And not only *can* you do it, with a little help from this book, you *will* do it.

When you succeed, we'd love to hear about it. So once *You Can Be as Young as You Think* has made a difference in your life, or if you have some youthful wisdoms of your own to pass on, please send us an email at: chris@ futurescoaching.com

And do visit we-rejuvenate.blogspot.com

01

The best-kept secret of staying young

We all want to stay young. We all want to be bright and inter-esting, to have plenty of energy and to relish life.

The scary thing is that some of us start to age in our thought patterns very early in life. This premature mental ageing process may pass almost unnoticed at first. It was Leo Tolstoy who said that 'the most surprising thing that happens to people is old age'. But the figures speak for themselves.

Just look at the statistics in the following table, drawn from a major study of British social attitudes,[1] broken down by age.

I am always searching for new things

	15–17	18–24	25–34	35–44	45–54	55–64	65+
% Agree	68	66	46	39	35	32	19

Source: Sociovision 3SC UK, 2005

[1] The data are drawn from a nationally representative sample of 1,800 British respondents and reproduced by kind permission of Sociovision, a well-established sociocultural research institute. Incidentally, regarding this data and all other statistical tables quoted in this book, a similar French study by Sociovision gave similar patterns by age bracket.

If you are aged over 25 this is a real wake-up call – you may be turning off already from the excitement of the new. In fact, one-fifth of 25–34 year olds are less likely to be searching for new things than they were in their late teens and early twenties.

Why is this important? For one, losing interest in novelty means losing a buzz from your life. More importantly, turning your back on the new means that your ability to embrace change will be so much more limited. And if you find change hard, life will become increasingly difficult.

We'll come across other data as we go through the book, and you'll get to see how this decline into Old Brain thinking crosses many dimensions of life. In a similar way, we'll reveal that the fall-off from youthful thinking starts extraordinarily early in most people's lives.

Return to the table above as we look at the other end of the age spectrum. As we see, there are 19 per cent of British people past the age of 65 who are still searching for new things. As time passes, they manage to remain interested, interesting and informed – vital and relevant. They are timeless. They are the lucky few.

For most of us, the feelings of getting old can start relatively early in life; aches and pains become more apparent by the day and 'senior moment' memory lapses ('Where did I put my keys?' 'Why did I come into this room?') begin sooner than most imagine. Mentally, we age by default. At some point we start wondering if we've lost touch with what life's all about. We don't laugh as much as we used to and generally we feel a bit tired, out of touch, somehow more grumpy – even wondering if we've run out of new and interesting things to say.

Rest assured: if you are worried about getting older you are not alone. Most of us have a morbid fascination with the subject. For the first 20 years of our lives we want to be older and for the remainder we aspire to be younger – until the day of reckoning when we have no more days left.

The warning signs of ageing may be all around you. Perhaps you've found at work that it is the younger members of the team who have all the bright ideas, and have the energy to realise them. Suddenly they start being promoted over your head. Or maybe you're still young in terms of years, but you find some of the older people at work more plugged in, more relevant – and, yes, younger than you in terms of outlook and performance. At home, it may be that your children are starting to gain greater independence of mind, leaving you feeling less useful and less tuned in to their wavelength.

Ironically, and despite all this clear evidence to the contrary, we can end up ignoring the warning signs of ageing and our age-related fallibilities. We dupe ourselves to protect our self-image. We like to push ageing out of mind in the hope that it will go away. The result is that ageing has a mischievous way of creeping up on us. Getting old happens to other people, you protest, not to me. I still feel myself to be 23!

And yet one day you find, almost unwittingly, that your attitudes have changed. You've become more negative, more pessimistic, less alert and somehow old at heart.

So, ask yourself the following questions:

● Do you still see the future as an exciting opportunity or has it become a foreign and inhospitable land? Have you ever told yourself, for example, that the future will be much bleaker than today?

● Are you already beginning to shut down on your hopes, your dreams and your desire to have fun?

● However young you are, have you started to separate yourself from the rest of society because of your age? For example, do you say things like: 'At my age, I'm not sure that's suitable?' Or 'I would have done it if I were younger'?

● Have you already had that heart-stopping moment when you hear yourself repeating your parents' phrases and suddenly you realise that you are becoming your father or your mother?

In defence of ageing

But wait a minute. In some senses, there is nothing wrong with getting older. It is entirely natural and can be highly dignified. We get to decide how late we stay out and what time we go to bed. We choose who and what we want in our lives. Hopefully we become more comfortable financially and, more importantly, comfortable with who we are.

Moreover, you would hope that more years on this earth brings more wisdom. This is wisdom won from reflection and from gaining sound judgement based on the lessons life teaches.

As a 30-year-old, it is rather heartening for one to believe that all the awkwardnesses of early human relationships are a thing of the past. And, by the time you are 40, it's fantastic to imagine that your stumbling mistakes as a gauche employee are behind you.

For many of us, the great comfort that accompanies the ageing process is the feeling that we have become more equipped for life's challenges and simply better at living our lives. Things that used to stress us are now dismissed as less important. There are fewer embarrassing situations; errors and faux pas become less frequent. The real meaning of life is discovered and embraced. Who could possibly want to be younger when maturity yields so much?

Here we must both agree and disagree.

We agree that it is entirely possible to learn vital lessons as we progress through life – learning what helps guide us to wiser choices. We refer to this as the 'wisdom of experience' and, in the last chapter of this book, we will argue that, taken together with the Wisdom of Youth, these two sources of wisdom will help you live a very rich and rewarding life indeed.

Where we disagree is with the general delusion that we all become sages as we progress through life's stages. For, while many people may think that they are accumulating wisdom, in reality they are often just amassing rigidity and pomposity. For these people, age brings little new learning. And as we shall see, on the contrary, that many people are more likely to be losing life skills over time than gaining them. Therefore, we need to challenge the assumption that, as we grow older, our bodies go into decline but our minds become rich and mellow.

'There is an assumption that as we get older we will get wiser; not true I'm afraid. The rule is we carry on being just as daft, still making plenty of mistakes. It's just that we make new ones, different ones.'

Richard Templar, *The Rules of Life*

'Experience is that marvellous thing that enables you to recognise a mistake when you make it again.'

F.P. Jones

A final defence that is often made of ageing is that it gets you off the hook. It gives you an alibi to avoid doing all those things you really don't want to do.

A 30-year-old happy-to-be-single woman might yearn to become 50 years old so that people would stop asking her when she will settle down, find a husband and start a family. She wishes neither to wed nor to have children, and being middle-aged would give her the perfect excuse not to be bothered about explaining these things.

This works for 65-year-olds just as easily. Yes, you might be a little more decrepit – but the good news is that people now don't make so many demands on you. Maybe you can even revel in the new status of the 'grumpy old wo/man', always reactionary – and often mildly entertaining to your entourage.

Unfortunately, while this 'slow-slide-into-senility' strategy has been valid across the decades, it is much less valid today. The simple truth is that ageing isn't what it used to be.

The need to be younger, older

Even three decades back, a slow descent into crabby thinking was possibly acceptable, even somewhat humorous. But today's dynamic society is becoming far less forgiving of yesteryear mentalities.

Nowadays, social pressure to live life to the full means that society is overthrowing the previously accepted stereotypes of ageing. Fifty is the new 30. Seventy is the new 50. Eighty is the new 60. Social pressure means that, for many, the idea that you can just relax and grow old gracefully increasingly is a thing of the past. Peer group pressure means middle-aged and elderly people have to be a lot more sprightly – and for a lot longer.

Of course, we are not saying that everyone, no matter what age, has to be tearing around like a teenager. It is entirely under-standable, as you get older, to want to replace, for example, vigorous or dangerous physical sports with less strenuous activities. Or to appreciate a night curled up by the fire as much as you once appreciated full-on all-night partying. Our point is that, today, people have both the opportunities and the social expectations to continue to grow throughout their lives. The simple truth is that not playing by these new rules can lead to personal frustration and possible lack of fulfilment.

Now, you might still take issue with us that, even in today's go-getter society, it is still possible to wind down over your life and gradually take your foot off the accelerator. To persuade you that this course of action is more problematic than it once was, let's take three examples.

The first is the change within families concerning attitudes to age. Only a couple of generations ago, sons wanted to be like their fathers and daughters like their mothers. Today, the evol-ution of social values means that roles have almost entirely reversed. Fathers want to be like their sons and mothers like their daughters. They shop together, buy similar 'young' clothes, listen to the same music, go to the same places. And, as the generations have blurred, society's expectations of older people have changed. You can no longer hide behind your age when attitude counts for so much. You are only as old as you think you are.

Second is the Viagra phenomenon. Only a few years ago, impotency brought on by ageing was generally accepted as the start of a slow decline in sexual appetite and activity. Today, however, the heat is on, so to speak. Can't perform? Then follow the example of millions of men, get down to the doctor's and do something about it. The opportunity to avoid a drooping libido exists, so why wouldn't you want to take advantage? Age is no excuse. Ageing men must arise!

You see how quickly an 'opportunity' can become almost an obligation. Once something such as Viagra comes along, mental attitudes cannot spring back to the era where it did not exist.

For the third illustration, let's look at the social expectations placed on older people. The British political leader Sir Menzies Campbell was hounded from office in 2007 principally because of the impression he gave of being overly old. Seeing and listening to him on television, he came across as an old man. Cartoons of a toothless Ming hobbling about with a Zimmer frame, and jokes in Parliament about his being hard of hearing led, ultimately, to his downfall. And he was only in his sixties at the time. The message, like it or not, is clear. Be youthful, or else!

It's not only society's expectations that have changed. With increases in life expectancy, it's a striking thought that if you're 40 years old today, statistically speaking, you have about half your life ahead of you. So it makes sense to get in some sort of shape to make those years as youthful and enjoyable as possible.

More to the point, it makes no sense at all to become out of touch with society for decades to come. Your best chance of keeping up with modern life is to develop a youthful mindset.

Now, chances are you've picked up this book because you instinctively realise most of this. You not only want to stay young, relevant, useful and active, but you understand that it is preferable to do so. Probably, you already suspect that a gradual decline into slippers and a rocking chair is not for you. You know that if you want to stay meaningfully engaged in life, you simply have to be ready and willing, as the phrase goes, 'to be a player'. Whether you are 25, 45 or even 75, it's game on!

This book is here to help you achieve your ambitions to stay youthful by revealing the best-kept secret of staying young. But before we tell all, let's briefly look at other, more common, anti-ageing strategies and discover why, at best, these are half-hearted compromises.

The limits of conventional anti-ageing strategies

A key message of this book is that, while most conventional anti-ageing strategies can have positive effects, they miss the point. Since mental ageing can start in the twenties, adopting anti-ageing strategies later in life may be like locking the stable door after the horse has bolted. If the mind has aged, remedial work on the body will be lopsided.

Let's look at the various conventional strategies.

Looking young through cosmetic makeovers is, well, just that – cosmetic. Not only that but the whole premise is built on wishful thinking – a delusion. Ask any woman to be truthful about, say, anti-wrinkle cream and she may tell you that she has real doubts about its efficacy but she *wants* to believe in it. It's about hope rather than reality. It's also about kidding yourself that you are doing something and that physical ageing is negotiable. The pity is that, by believing this dream, you are diverting your attention from the very strategies that can help you rejuvenate sustainably.

Meanwhile, the surgical make-overs that allow people to buy their own slice of Hollywood glamour are also highly problematical. For a start, results are very often only temporary. Injecting Botox is a six-monthly cycle for the rest of your life. More crucially, investing to look physically younger counts for little if you remain old in the head. What good is Adonis when you think like old Uncle Alfred? Your sex appeal lasts just so long as you don't open your mouth. Can there be anything more embarrassing than attracting the attention of a younger person only to see him or her turn away when your real age is betrayed by your stuck-in-the-mud values and opinions. Your cover is well and truly blown. The danger is that you end up with a fabulous body and a frumpy brain.

While we would be the last to discourage working out and eating well, these strategies are only the foundations; they also do not go far enough in helping you live a young life. They will certainly help you live longer, but the most effective strategy combines quantity with quality.

What about the mind-sharpening exercises? Suduku and crossword puzzles are good, but they may mean we are simply quicker at saying or doing something that is intrinsically old-fashioned or out of phase with the times. Mental exercises are unlikely to prevent us from turning into a grumpy old man or woman. They won't help us keep up with trends and events – or stop us becoming outdated. So sharpening the saw is good, but it's still a halfway house.

Doing young things is not guaranteed to roll back the years either. Acting young can be beneficial, of course, but with old values and opinions racing around your brain, how rejuvenating can this really be?

Take the traveller to far-off places. Adventurousness is highly commendable but it is not the whole story. If it isn't accompanied by an ability to learn about other cultures it does little to rejuvenate the mind. Two weeks touring the Caribbean on a luxury cruise liner is unlikely to reduce your mental age.

In short, ageing is insidious and can affect us physically, mentally and psychologically at a profound level. In the face of this reality, creams, crosswords and Caribbean cruises are akin to re-arranging the deckchairs on the Titanic.

The truth is that if you really want a youthful life, and the success and happiness that goes with it, you must adopt a totally different rejuvenation strategy.

The secret of staying young: mindset change

The authentic elixir isn't to be found with lotions, breast implants, word puzzles or outings to pop concerts. These are quick-fix solutions that give a veneer of youth, no more. The real secret to staying young is to develop and retain a youthful mindset. Put another way, achieving the dream of enduring youth is about changing the way you think.

Youth is no longer a demographic; it is a state of mind. It is not a matter of rosy cheeks and kissable lips. It is about the quality of imagination, the vigour of emotions and the will to action.

To be young you must think young. You must set aside the cranky thoughts and re-establish the attitudes, values and sharp thought patterns of young people.

Moreover, to be young you must also be relevant, up to date, in contact with the changes in the world around you. The mindset change that we recommend is also about thinking modern thoughts, aligned with modern progress. It's about being in touch and in the flow. It's about embodying values and opinions that minimise the dissonance between your perspectives and today's society. It's about altering the way you think about our ever-evolving world and abandoning prejudice and fear as you go.

'Staying young is a state of mind ... not being reactionary or being disapproving of more and more things, not settling for what you've always had or always done.'

Richard Templar, *The Rules of Life*

This is a double whammy. As we unveil the Wisdom of Youth, we will introduce you to both young thinking and relevant thinking.

Finally, when we speak about mindset change, we speak about something quite fundamental. Once thought patterns are deeply embedded and repeated naturally, we can then talk about a changed personality. By thinking youthful thoughts and, by consequence, engaging in genuinely youthful behaviours, people become young. Period.

'You are as young as your faith, as old as your doubt; as young as your self-confidence, as old as your fears; as young as your hope, as old as your despair. In the central place of every heart, there is a recording chamber; so long as it receives messages of beauty and hope, cheer and courage, you are young. When the wires are all down and your heart is covered with the snows of pessimism and the ice of cynicism, then and only then, have you grown old.'

General MacArthur

As we've already said, the truth is that some people manage to stay young without much effort. They have been blessed with a personality that remains forever young. The Wisdom of Youth that they were born with never seems to leave them. They are happy-go-lucky, spontaneous, have lots of friends of whatever age and energy to spare.

Others, and you may be one of them, have personalities that seem to age more quickly. Such is life.

But the important point is not from where you are starting from but where you are going. This should come as a huge relief to you. You *can* take control of your life and you *can* rejuvenate. If you have become old before your time, it is probably because you've not retained the Wisdom of Youth. This book is your chance to remodel your life.

And let's not forget – you deserve to be youthful and dynamic. You deserve everything that is magical, exciting and marvellous about life. We all do. It just requires the motivation and effort to change. And the moment to make changes has never been better than **NOW!**

The right stuff

But how do you change mindsets and rejuvenate? The surprisingly simple answer is by rediscovering the Wisdom of Youth. Basically, we are asking you to do no more than reclaim what you may have been losing en route.

Ah! But you say, there are some rather unseemly aspects of extreme youth as well. I also lost those en route. I don't want to roll back the years only to find myself feeling awkward or rebellious or antisocial. My youthful mindset was not always wise – or wholesome for that matter!

That is an important point and this book hinges on clarifying the key issue. We are absolutely not suggesting that you adopt, hook line and sinker, all the values and behaviours of today's young people. That would be reckless. Our thrust is to invite you to take what is best about youth; those mindsets that allow you to rediscover how to live contemporary life easily and richly. These wholesome facets are what we call the Wisdom of Youth.

As for the rest of youth – the follies, the self-obsession, the ungrateful attitudes, the transgression (not to mention the pimples) – we'll leave all those well behind.

It is also vital that we say, up front, that we thoroughly sub-scribe to the idea that, at least for some, ageing does bring new wisdom. We will go some way to address the 'wisdom of expe-rience' in the final chapter. However, our main theme is youthful wisdom – an overlooked phenomenon and one that some readers might even think paradoxical. We will focus most of our attention here.

Now, while we pause momentarily to be clear on definitions, let's come back to two terms that we've already started to use: 'Young Brain' and 'Old Brain'. We'll be referring time and again to these two concepts as the book unfolds. So it's worth being clear about exactly what we mean.

When we mention Young Brains we are referring to people who have retained the Wisdom of Youth in their lives – and, signifi-cantly, have discarded the follies of youth. But please note that a Young Brain is not necessarily young in years. Here's the good news. You can have a Young Brain at any age.

Old Brains, meanwhile, are people who have lost much of the Wisdom of Youth. In their rush to be respected as adults, they have discarded, all too rapidly, their younger selves. And, weighed down by their grown-up responsibilities, Old Brains have abandoned their youthful enthusiasm for life. Once again, you can have an Old Brain at almost any age – as you'll discover in the next chapter.

Young Brains therefore have the 'right stuff' – and so should you. The key to sustainable rejuvenation is to think like a Young Brain and perpetuate the Wisdom of Youth.

By taking objective social science research and re-analysing the data, we have uncovered and defined six wisdoms of youth. And the amazing thing is this. Despite the deceptively simple nature of our solution to ageing, this is a story only now being told. It's a secret between you and us.

So, having picked up *You Can Be as Young as You Think* and got this far, you should pat yourself on the back. For you are holding in your hands something rather powerful. Used correctly, the Six Steps we will unfold in Chapters 3–8 will allow you to stay younger and feel sharper.

Can there be anything more exciting than that?

02

So, just how old are you?

Birthdays, body age and brain age

Most people understand that there is a difference between chronological age and physiological age. Our chronological age is simply the number of birthdays we've had. Our physiological age – or 'body age' – is how a doctor might assess the age of your organs, bones and skin. For example, if you are young but a heavy smoker, you will have 'old' lungs. There can be many years difference between your birthdays and your body age.

Then there's brain age. Your brain age is the age of your mindset, your mental approach to life. Do you have a Young Brain, an Old Brain or something in between? This is measured, not by doctors, nor by arithmetic puzzles but by social scientists. We'll be asking you to take a brain age test in just a moment.

Surprisingly, our brain's age may bear even less relevance to the numbers of birthdays we've notched up than our body age.

So, no one grows old by merely living a number of years. People grow old by not looking after their bodies and, importantly, by deserting the instinctive wisdom of their early years.

Our three ages can all be different and usually are. For example, following is the profile of John Fossil:

Birthdays: 55	Body age: 45	Brain age 63

John is 55 years old and is physically fit. But he has the mindset of a 63-year-old. You've probably met him – he's the sort of person who is into exercise but not into thinking. His body moves well, but his mind is pretty static.

Now meet Janey Tack:

Birthdays: 63	Body age: 52	Brain age 35

Janey has a body age, and particularly a brain age, which is some way short of her chronological age. She is mentally sharp and very young at heart. You've probably met her too. Evergreen, she's plugged in to today's world, full of enthusiasm for life, and can talk to anyone – particularly children – as equals.

And here's Jimmy McFogey:

Birthdays: 29	Body age: 33	Brain age 41

Jimmy's body age is close to his birthdays – he understands the importance of a healthy body and works out regularly. The trouble is, his attitudes and mindset are inward-looking, defensive and anxious. He doesn't expect too much joy and excitement in life, and doesn't find it.

As we saw in Chapter 1, the most important discriminator of age isn't body age, still less birthdays; it's your brain's age. Many people are 'old' because they have 'old' mindsets. They have 'old' ways of looking at things. Their perceptions and insights are less meaningful in today's society. They have out-of-date ideas. They have Old Brains. And this matters.

'Success often depends on the relative age of your ideas. And today, people of all ages are in trouble because their ideas aren't just old, they're obsolete'

Robert Kiyosaki, author of *Rich Dad, Poor Dad*

Establish your Youth Quotient by taking the Brain Age Test

So what age is your brain? Or put another way, what is your YQ – or Youth Quotient? There is only one way to find out and that's by testing yourself with our Brain Age Test.

The Brain Age Test draws on robust research from the social sciences to provide a measurement of your brain's YQ. Not in terms of how quickly you can do mental arithmetic or complete a difficult crossword, but in terms of your mindset.

There are 12 questions you need to answer by choosing one of the three options offered. We should say that, in setting this test, we have assumed that you wish to draw maximum value out of this book. We have not tried, therefore, to disguise the Brain Age Test and it may be pretty obvious where most of the questions are leading. Although it may be tempting to give answers that make your thinking appear younger than it currently is, DON'T GIVE IN TO THE TEMPTATION.

BE HONEST. Give rapid, spontaneous answers that describe what you would actually think or do. Honesty will avoid depriving yourself of the opportunity to gain some genuine insights that, in turn, will spur you on to make changes in your life.

Incidentally, the questions you will be answering cover some of the key values linked to ageing, i.e. the various statements are highly discriminating by age. In answering them honestly, the results will reveal something about your personality and beliefs. Your responses will show what you attach importance to in your life today and, consequently, locate the age of your thinking within a specific age cohort.

It is important to understand that brain age as a concept involves no judgements on morality. It does not say some values are morally good and some are morally bad. Nevertheless, it does involve taking a view about our values. It says some values are younger and more relevant to the world we live in, and some are less so.

By completing the Brain Age Test, you'll have a view on your current YQ. This is a snapshot in time. At the end of the book we'll invite you to take the test again, once you've had a chance to ingest the Wisdom of Youth. The aim, of course, is that by reading this book and by following through, there will be a measurable increase in you YQ.

Here goes. Good luck.

The Brain Age Test

1 You receive a personal invitation to join a crowd of people for a social day out. You know these people only vaguely. Do you:

   a Make your excuses and refuse the invite?

   b Accept on the condition that you can invite someone you know well (your partner, close friend, etc.)?

   c Say you'd love to come as you often have a good time in crowds?

2 While at a wedding, a group of children ask if you would like to have a go with a skipping rope. Do you:

   a Say no, as you will crease and dirty your wedding outfit?

   b Offer to hold one end of the rope while one of the children skips?

   c Jump at the chance to rediscover your child within?

3 You find yourself being pressurised to give up more of your spare time than you can sensibly spare for a good cause. Do you reply:

   a It's my duty to serve others so, of course, I'll put in the extra time?

   b I need to keep balance in my life, so I'll do it for a while and then we'll see?

   c In order to operate effectively, it's important that I also help myself, so I cannot accept the extra work?

4 Faced with the launch of a new electrical gadget, what is your reaction:

a I wait and see. Once it's been tried and tested by others, I might then buy it?

b I judge it on its merits, looking carefully at the benefits and whether it would be useful to me?

c If it looks interesting, I'll buy it and have a play; you never know until you try?

5 How would you *best* describe the personality you cultivate in *public*? Are you:

a Very professional, strait-laced and constant over time?

b Someone with a strong sense of ethics and social justice?

c Rather informal and playful; an amusing actor on the stage of life?

6 Thinking about education and personal development, are you:

a At ease with what you've been taught; there's no need to learn any more?

b Enthusiastic about self-development, getting involved in things such as adult education and often reading serious books?

c A 'sponge' who learns instinctively and is forever questioning why things are the way they are?

7 'It is important to lead a life full of entertainment, excitement and risk.' How far do you agree?:

a I disagree with this statement; life is much more serious than this.

b I tend to agree; life is there to be enjoyed.

c I strongly agree with this; it's important to get the most out of life.

8 How do you react when things go wrong and your best-laid plans are in danger of being scuppered? Do you:

a Become frustrated and stubborn?

b Find who or what is responsible and sort things out with them?

c Go with the flow; a change of direction is only to be expected?

9 Thinking about people and institutions in general, over the last three years or so, would you say that you've become:

a More sceptical of others?

b Ready to give others the benefit of the doubt?

c More trusting of others?

10 Imagine you had a difficult decision to take regarding your future. How would you take that decision:

a Using only rational considerations?

b Listen to you feelings but then try to decide rationally?

c Give full reign to gut feel, trying to decide instinctively what's the right thing to do?

11 You know a teenager who is a real dreamer. How do you react:

a You advise him or her to 'wake up' and get his or her feet firmly on the ground?

b You don't interfere; people are who they are.

c You strongly encourage him or her; dreams, imagination and an artistic temperament should be cultivated in people?

12 When you go grocery shopping, do you:

   a Pick out the brands and products that you have always bought?

   b Carefully choose between brands and products that are right for you?

   c Experiment with unknown brands and newly launched products?

Discovering your Brain Age

Now's the time to discover if you have a Young Brain, an Old Brain or something in-between.

Finding out your YQ is very simple. For those questions where you have answered 'a' give yourself 1 point; 'b' gets you 2 points; and for answer 'c' give yourself 3 points. Add your points to give a sum total and find your Youth Quotient in the ranges below. Within any given range, next look for your chronological age to correctly understand what your results are telling you.

YQ of 12–18 points: Old Brain

Most of your answers were a's and b's indicating that your brain thinks like an old person thinks.

If you have passed your 65th birthday: although your brain age is in alignment with your chronological age, you are far from benefiting from the Wisdom of Youth. Life is steady, predictable and winding down. You probably feel out of touch with others outside your peer group and fearful of the changes you see around you.

If you are between 45 and 65 years old: you are old before your time. Adopt the Wisdom of Youth – and forget the anti-ageing creams and sudoku until you've done something about your mindset.

If you are under 45 years old: unless you have chosen to be an old fogey, this is a worrying finding. You are probably out of step with most of your friends and peers, and prefer the company of older generations. You'll have the feeling that others are passing you on the road while you are dawdling on the inside lane. There is a very real danger that introversion will cut you off from others and from leading a fulfilling life.

YQ of 19–29 points: Middle-aged Brain

You will have chosen lots of b's or have a fairly even spread from 1–3. Your brain thinks and acts like it's middle-aged.

If you have passed your 65th birthday: you have a younger YQ than your chronological age and have certain values that you share with younger generations. Although you have resisted a headlong slide into the thought patterns of Old Brains, you can still benefit from the Wisdom of Youth.

If you are between 45 and 65 years old: your brain age matches your chronological age. You will find lots of common ground with the majority of your peers but you also find that younger generations are different and perplexing. You sometimes find yourself wondering if you've let something rather precious slip from your grasp as you've got older. You have. You've lost the Wisdom of Youth.

If you are under 45 years old: you are old before your time. You should have youthful wisdom and boldness on your side but instead you have latched on to middle-aged thoughts, feelings and behaviours. You may want to ask yourself what has happened along the way to accelerate your brain's ageing process?

YQ of 30–36 points: Young Brain

You will have answered with mostly cs and a few bs, indicating a Young Brain.

If you have passed your 65th birthday: people call you 'evergreen'. You have good relationships with younger generations and with your grandchildren, if you have them. You identify with today's society and its changes and are probably still involved in creating and leading those changes. Maybe you are still working or very active in a number of associations or in the community. The Wisdom of Youth is yours – but reading on will help explain why you are the way you are and ensure you stay that way.

If you are between 45 and 65 years old: you have not rested on your laurels and continue to put yourself to the test. Not for you the gentle slide into middle age; you continue to move with the times and probably have good relationships with younger generations including, if you have them, your children. The insights of the Wisdom of Youth in the forthcoming chapters will help ensure you keep up your guard and stay fresh.

If you are under 45 years old: you are young and you think young. Being aligned with your generation and with the latest social changes, you are ideally positioned to exploit everything life has to offer you. Positive, energetic and versatile, you epitomize the Wisdom of Youth. Read on to ensure that you never let slip from your grasp what comes naturally to you today.

What is your brain telling you?

Assuming you've been entirely honest in your answers and haven't gone for the younger-sounding options merely to feel better about yourself, you may have found that your YQ is a bit lower than you had hoped for and that, therefore, your brain is older than you'd imagined. If you did find yourself with an old or Middle-aged Brain, you are certainly not alone – the majority of people accept a slow and steady decline into senescent thinking.

But, if your brain is telling you that it's got itself old, how much of a worry is this? In all honesty, it should be of real concern. Putting it in a nutshell, an Old Brain can both isolate you and stress you; it can make you more cynical and pessimistic about the future; it can be both limiting and divisive.

People with older brains tend to shut the doors on excitement, rejecting risk and avoiding challenge in the name of a 'quiet life'. An Old Brain hates novelty and works very hard to keep mental stimulation at bay. Dreams and imagination are potentially dangerous and should be subdued as quickly as possible.

Having an older brain also means avoiding things that are found trying or inconvenient, such as strangers, or friends-of-friends. Or, more debilitating still, questions. Questions can be provocative and require you to think about long-held opinions, or what you are doing and why. Questions are the enemy of the Old Brain. 'Things are as they are and let's leave it at that,' says the Old Brain. Not exactly the recipe for staying up with the times.

Neither is there room in an Old Brain's mindset for self-exploration. One's personality and psychology are best treated as a black box. Old Brains tend to ring-fence emotions and limit their impacts. Consequently, they inhibit the pleasure they take from life too.

On the other hand, if your brain is telling you that you have a high YQ – i.e. you have a Young Brain – good for you! But, now is not the time to rest on your laurels. By making the implicit Wisdom of Youth explicit, the rest of this book will help you avoid the pitfalls of ageing, help you steer clear of Old Brain thinking and consciously keep you the way you are.

Personal starting point

For the record, note the following:

My birthdays:

My YQ:

My Brain Age (old, middle-aged or young):

Date:

Now, be ambitious and set yourself a challenge:

My YQ goal:

Date:

Incidentally, we'll be referring to Young Brains throughout this book and contrasting them with older brains. For simplicity, we will not compare to both Old Brains and Middle-aged Brains every time we want to illustrate differences in mindsets. We will use only Old Brains as the point of comparison. If you have a Middle-aged Brain, your mindset is clearly between what we describe for Young Brains and for Old Brains.

SUMMARY

To summarise where we've got to so far:

- We've seen that youthfulness and ageing are two of the major issues of our times.

- We've understood that conventional anti-ageing strategies are partial and will not deliver the dream of enduring youth.

- We've learned that the best-kept secret of staying young is to change mindsets and think younger, more relevant thoughts.

- You've measured your starting YQ and understood the implications of your current brain age.

- You've set yourself a YQ target.

Over the next six chapters, we will:

- Meet the Six Steps to staying younger and feeling sharper – the wisdoms of youth.

- Describe each wisdom one by one and list the youthful benefits each wisdom brings.

- Look at the exact mindsets Young Brains deploy.

- Show you the very practical and achievable actions you can take to adopt these youthful mindsets.

- Summarise your rejuvenation goals.

Ready to change for ever? Let's go.

03

Adaptive Navigation

It was hot, and the passengers were angry. Their plane to Puerto Rico had been cancelled.

Most of them had been on vacation on the Caribbean island, but the holiday mood soon evaporated. Their anger slowly turned to sullen resignation. It would be a 24-hour delay. At least. They milled around, in the words of Robert Burns, 'nursing their wrath to keep it warm'.

Suddenly, one of the passengers emerged with a blackboard and chalked on it 'Virgin Airways. $39 single flight to Puerto Rico'. It was Richard Branson. He was one of the disappointed passengers on the charter flight but, rather than sit around fuming, he had chartered a plane for $2,000, and had then divided the sum by the number of passengers, which came to $39 a head. The idea that was to become Virgin Airways was born.

This is Adaptive Navigation in action. When plans are disrupted an Old Brain sits around and gets angry. A Young Brain says, 'Okay. The situation's changed. Let's find a way round it.'

Defining Adaptive Navigation

Adaptive Navigation is the term we use to describe the mindset which takes a flexible attitude to life's challenges and changes. Traditional approaches to life stress the idea of fixing a goal and then taking the most direct path towards it. However, this form of planning only works until life intervenes. In other words, when change happens it throws everything off course and can cause the original plan to be abandoned.

Adaptive Navigation represents a different approach. It still involves having an idea of where you want to get to, but it includes a heavy dose of realism. The method, then, is to set sail towards the objective but *be ready* to be blown off course. Then by 'tacking' into the wind, you correct for this chance factor and, once again head back towards your goal.

Adaptive Navigation requires skill, quick reactions and decisions but, above all, an openness to change. And, of course, this openness has never been more necessary than it is today.

Everyone knows that change happens and that it's happening faster and faster, but do you ever stop to think about what this really means? It's worth a quick reminder of just how much change you've actually witnessed in your life.

For a moment think back to the world of your childhood and remember the pace of life then. How quickly did messages get to you? Bear in mind that, if we go back merely 40 years, it was only the well-off minority that had a fixed-line telephone. Perhaps it took three days to receive a letter in the post, you took one day to write back and the correspondent received your reply in the post after another three days. Today you receive an email or text message immediately after it was sent, reply directly and the correspondent can have your answer in front of his or her eyes in a matter of seconds. MSN messaging and mobile phone texting have made the typed one-liner the new art of conversation: Cn u do it LOL.

Take another area of life – photography. Time was when a roll of film might stay in the camera for weeks or more. Remember that? Then, to process and develop it there was another wait. Several days later, you went to the shop and picked up 24 precious photos from last Christmas. Seems incredible now, doesn't it? Today, we are not talking about 24, but 240 pictures, and these can be viewed and edited on screen almost immediately after they are taken, and sent around the world a few seconds later.

We now have 200+ TV channels – not a mere two or three – and thousands of digital radio stations available from around the world rather than a handful from our local and national providers. Our supermarkets are stocked with over 50,000 different items versus around 10,000 of yesteryear. Certain supermarket chains introduce as many as 3,000 new lines in a single year. We could go on and on.

And the point is this. Change has affected our everyday lives much more that we think. Everything – products, organisations, situations – changes faster. So long-term planning for a fixed tomorrow is yesteryear's approach. Ducking, bobbing, weaving, thinking on your feet, navigating adaptively, these are the approaches that pay the highest dividends today.

So, the Young Brain understands that planning is important but, unlike the Old Brain, is not upset when things change and a rethink is required. Rather than get angry, the Young Brain response is 'No worries. Forget the plan.' Young Brains know that being open to, and excited by, change is more effective in producing health, wealth and fulfilment than holding on to constancy and stability at all costs.

Accepting the new

Now, we all like to think that we are open-minded and that we enjoy new situations. We see ourselves as up to date. We are interested in what is happening in the world and what is new. And this comfortable belief stays with us as we get older.

The facts, however, blow away our self-congratulation as a delusion. Only the young really embrace the new. Let's look again at the table we examined earlier:

I am always searching for new things

	15–17	18–24	25–34	35–44	45–54	55–64	65+
% Agree	68	66	46	39	35	32	19

Source: Sociovision 3SC UK, 2005

Yes, these figures are shocking. The fall-off in passion for new things starts remarkably early in our lives. The drums of Old Brain thinking start to beat almost as soon as we enter adulthood. That's a very scary thought!

This chapter is the big one. If you can get into the mindset of Adaptive Navigation and enjoy change, the other five wisdoms will fall into place more easily. If you find it difficult to change, the other chapters will be slightly harder going.

But, on the positive side, the essence of Adaptive Navigation – being light on planning and heavy on intuition and responsiveness – is an entirely reasonable goal. And you'll be relieved to hear that anyone can do it.

Be assured that we in no way underestimate the challenges involved. What may in this and the following chapters, sound a bit like tough love is just that – tough love. Some of the issues involving ageing brains and the loss of youthful wisdom need facing up to, and taking on the chin. We – and you – have to be honest in addressing the issues. There are things we all need to hear. If we pretend it's easy, we will be doing everyone a disservice, and possibly depriving you of the opportunity to improve your life.

The good news is you can do it – whether you are 30 or 70. As we showed in Chapter 1, what it requires is a shift in mindset. What this means is that the amount of improvement in your Youth Quotient is to a large degree dependent on how much you are willing to participate actively in both being open to the wisdoms of youth and taking the actions we recommend to help them become part of your thinking and behaviour.

Change is seldom easy, but if you have the courage to remould your life, and overcome the real or imagined obstacles that seem to loom in front of you, you can reap the substantial benefits of this first Wisdom of Youth.

Don't resist change

The Old Brain tends to fight change and, if it can, to reject it. Change is scary. It means leaving something safe behind. It means making an effort. It implies stretching yourself and taking personal risks. It can have unintended consequences on you and others around you. Thus, despite the seductive benefits of change, you may find yourself resisting this first Wisdom of Youth. It's natural to feel a bit panicked by invocations to change. We are tempting you into unknown and untested areas which you may have been sidestepping for years. However, the time has come to stop driving with one foot on the brake. By releasing the brake you'll find the journey more enjoyable and the scenery more interesting.

Unfortunately, Old Brains continue driving with their foot firmly on the brake pedal. They face two negative consequences.

The first is that they have a tendency to get particularly angry and frustrated at the values and behaviours they see around them. For example, they see the behaviour of the young as simply deplorable. This perception of the young is deeply unsettling, causing older people to feel both physically threatened and out of sync with the times they live in.

Old Brains conveniently forget what their own parents thought about their behaviour when they were young. And what their grandparents thought of their parents' before them.

'Every old man complains of the growing depravity of the world, and the petulance and insolence of the rising generation.'

Dr Samuel Johnson 1709–1784

In other words, there is nothing more unusual about the current vintage of younger person than any other time in history. Given this, Old Brains really are neither making a social nor ethical statement by cold-shouldering the young; they are simply leaving themselves out in the cold.

The second result of rejecting change is that Old Brains are missing out on a whole lot of enjoyment and satisfaction. It's a double whammy. They reject change, miss the benefits, and then get extremely angry when they see other people enjoying the fun.

Pushed to adapt to the spinning world, the Old Brain stands shoulder to shoulder with King Canute. It rails against the waves of change and resists them. The Young Brain says, 'Surf the waves.' And once you have increased your Youth Quotient, so will you.

The benefits of Adaptive Navigation

So what's in it for you? By applying a more adaptive approach to navigation you'll not only avoid these dual frustrations, you'll benefit from many positives. The following are some of the key ones:

- Planning is more realistic and liberated.
- Change happens and you can benefit. You'll be grateful not fearful.
- Engaging in new situations leads to a lot more fun.
- Being back in tune, intuitively, with how things work.

- Widening your comfort zone, meaning more different experiences to enjoy; less embarrassment, more excitement.

- Avoiding negative rearguard actions that are doomed to failure.

- Replacing lots of old stuff that no longer really works for products, services and ideas, offering innovative solutions to daily problems.

- Improving relationships with the opposite sex.

- Discovering your unexpected talents.

- Participating more authentically in the lives of your children and grandchildren.

- Waking up to some of society's future challenges and being ready to play your part.

- Finally, a feeling of being alive; no more sleepwalking through life.

In order to enjoy these benefits of Adaptive Navigation, there are three key actions to take.

1 Be prepared to give up comfort zones

2 Open yourself to values realignment

3 Adopt the three change mindsets of Young Brains

Let's take these one at a time.

Be prepared to give up comfort zones

It's important to understand that in the early days of being open to change you are likely to be right outside your comfort zone. Don't worry. As you do more of it, the scary stuff gets to be easier, and fun. You'll get better and better at it, and wonder how you did without the huge stimulus change can bring in so many areas of your life.

This is true whether you are 30, 60 or 90, because if you want to benefit from the Wisdom of Youth, and open up the exciting potential of a young, engaged brain, it may require that you face up to the fear of losing these protective havens. Let's look at a selection of comfort zones you may have been settling into, without realising just how much they are insulating you from the realities of the world at large:

- The reassuring belief that your opinions are right, and the only ones a sensible person would hold (without giving up this one, mindset change will be very challenging).
- A belief that the way you do things is the right way.
- A carefully (and possibly unconsciously) built-up belief that you are in some way superior to other people (more successful, privileged or personable).
- A belief in the old certainties of wealth, class and education.
- A belief in the importance of the position/authority you have in your workplace/family/home.
- A sense of financial superiority (size of car/house).
- A feeling that the old ways are the best ways.
- The idea that the young have nothing to offer and everything to learn.
- The notion that as you get older you always get wiser.
- The conviction that if you just hunker down and avoid making any changes, you can avoid bad things happening in your life.

Starting to widen your comfort zones

If you are nestling in one or two – or more – of these comfort zones, don't worry. We understand. We've all been there. Our message is simple, however. You will increase your chances for success in life – and your enjoyment of it – if you are prepared to change.

Comfort thinking is a bit like sweet and fatty comfort food. It feels warm and pleasurable at the time, but you tend to pay the price later when your arteries or, in the case of comfort thinking, your neural pathways start to clog up.

So here is a list of actions you might take to start to ease yourself out of the mental comfort zones you may have unwittingly settled into:

- Start to ask *'Why not?'* when faced with different ways of doing things, instead of giving an immediate 'No'.
- Faced with a new or challenging situation, ask yourself if there might be a different or better way to deal with it than your immediate, preprogrammed, response.
- Start to look for the benefits or advantages in the ways other people do things or respond to situations.
- Ask questions of everyone about everything – you'll be surprised what you learn.
- Ask yourself questions, such as 'What if I were wrong about this'? Start being more humble.
- Try giving people the benefit of the doubt when they do things in a different way from you.
- Start to trust other people more – chances are they are not being intentionally perverse or stupid.
- Try varying the newspapers and magazines that you read and the TV you watch, to get some different viewpoints on what's really going on in the world.

Comfort zones hold us captive – but also make us a vulnerable sitting duck. Change makes us a safer moving target and more interesting as well. So cut those restraining ropes and start to fly.

Be open to values realignment

What we are talking about here is being ready to update your perspectives, values, attitudes and, consequently, your behaviour so you can be more in sympathy with your surroundings. Some changes may be significant, others may be small but important tweaks, and still others will be reappraisals and re-interpretations. Once you are more in alignment with what is going on around you, you'll find life less stressful (you'll be a lot less grumpy for starters), more enjoyable and more satisfying. It's a profound wisdom, and one worth working at to rediscover.

At this point it's quite possible you're thinking something along the lines of: Change my *values*? The very idea! But please, please take a deep breath and trust us on this one. We will not be asking you to do anything immoral. Uncomfortable, possibly, but immoral – no.

When you start out, re-evaluating deeply held values may take some digestion. Changing or adapting values, attitudes and behaviours goes to the core of who you are as a person, so you will need to tread carefully.

The first thing to do is to find out about your current values.

To do this, think through, and then set down on paper, a list of ten principles or values you hold dearest to your heart. This is not a five-minute job, but it's important. Don't put it off till later. If you need help with this, try visiting Tim Drake's website www.iwanttomakeadifference.com and look at the Tools/Values Map drop-downs.

The Following is a list of some values taken from the website – there are lots more there to mull over at your leisure. This list, however, may help to quickstart your thinking on this:

Achievement	Fame	Openness
Accountability	Fidelity	Personal development
Adventure	Family	Planning
Affection	Financial security	Pleasure
The arts	Freedom	The past
Autonomy	Free enterprise	The present
Being the best	Fulfilment	Quality
Being right	Fun	Recognition
Business building	Giving	Reliability
Capitalism	Goodness	Religion
Caring	Happiness	Respect
Celebrity	Honesty	Responsibility
Challenge	Health	Responsiveness
Civic	Iconoclasm	Security
responsibilities		
Civil liberties	Inclusiveness	Self-control
Competence	Independence	Service
Conservation	Individual	Self-esteem
	responsibility	
Consistency	Initiative	Spontaneity
Cooperation	Integrity	Spirituality
Control	Justice	Tidiness
Culture	Humour	Tradition
Connecting with	Leadership	Trust
people		
Enthusiasm	Learning	Volunteering
Excellence	Love	Winning
Fairness	Loyalty	Wisdom

Picking ten from this lot isn't easy. Most of them look attractive and worthwhile. The point is that you are trying to get a closer fix on exactly who you are and what you stand for. What is really important to you? What gets your juices going, and defines your essential distinctiveness as a human being?

Once you have decided on your top ten values, put them in priority order. This too can be challenging, as all your top ten will look important and worthwhile. But persevere, because once you know your top three or four values, you will start to get an insight into what motivates you at a profound level.

The vital thing to understand about the list is that *your values will – and should – change over time*. Don't be concerned about this – it's natural. Indeed it's the crux of being able to change mindset and adopt the Wisdom of Youth. In fact, if you do adopt the Wisdom of Youth, your list may have changed by the end of this book. And certainly by the end of the year. If values drop off your list, it doesn't mean they are unimportant, just that more important ones have taken over.

As an example, following is a list of the top ten values that someone might embrace now. Your own list will probably be very different – indeed it might be interesting to compare your list with this one before you move on.

Example: today's top ten values
Family
Caring
Honesty
Reliability
Loyalty
Recognition
Fulfilment
Control
Civic responsibilities
Respect

These are all positive, worthwhile values, and define the person holding them as being a good and caring citizen, keen to put something back into society. This is who the person is now: their life has meaning and their values indicate a life well lived.

Applying the lessons throughout this book – and working on the lessons having read it – could lead to that person's values shifting over time. His or her values might evolve into looking something like this:

Example: top ten values after reading book
Family
Caring
Fun
Fufilment
Enthusiasm
Openness
Connecting
Giving
Responsiveness
Recognition

It's the same person, but his or her values have evolved over time as they have taken on board the Wisdom of Youth. They still retain many of their own values – family and caring, for instance – but values such as fun and openness have increased in importance.

Before taking on board the insights into how he or she could increase his or her Youth Quotient, chances are that fun and openness wouldn't have figured in their top 20 or 30, let alone their top ten values. At the same time, reliability and control have become less important for them, as other more vibrant youthful values have taken over.

Let's be clear. We are not suggesting for one moment that you should be open to, or adopt, all change. Some change is good, some is neutral, some is bad and some is downright dangerous.

If the change you are examining is contrary to all you hold dear, in fact it is morally repellent, then, of course, refuse it outright.

What we are suggesting is that *you look for the good in change*.

From now on, carefully and unemotionally examine developments in society's values as they cross your radar screen for acceptability on a moral basis (i.e. does it conflict with your principles?). If you accept that there's no or little conflict, go with the flow. Make that change in your life – from today.

Adopt three Adaptive Navigation mindsets as your own

Once you have done this necessary groundwork, you can move on to the first major step of improving your Youth Quotient by thinking younger and sharper.

That step is to adopt a new approach to organising and planning your life.

Since Adaptive Navigation is all about making changes in your life, we need start to reprogramme your old or Middle-aged Brain with three Young Brain mindsets:

1 Living a 'Lite Life'

2 Taking Street Savvy decisions

3 Gender Blending

This means looking at the what, the how, and the who. **What** you change will be down to your planning, and Young Brains have an approach we call 'Lite Life'. **How** you change comes down to your decision-making. The Young Brain approach is to take 'Street Savvy' decisions. Finally, **who** does what is about assigning roles and responsibilities. The Young Brain has a flexible, rolling view of how tasks are allocated and 'Gender Blend' is a good description of this functioning within a couple.

Everyone can change, and so can you. If you find yourself clinging to Old Brain values, these three Young Brain mindsets (Lite Life, Street Savvy and Gender Blending) will help you to rejuvenate. And remember, these are the tried and tested approaches used by Young Brains. If you feel as if you're being overtaken in life, simply place Adaptive Navigation at the heart of your thinking. We'll show you how. Just follow the actions we suggest after each box headed 'Living the Wisdom'.

1. Living a 'Lite Life'

We all have comfort zones. Sometimes they are discomfort zones. Like a dog lying on a sharp and uneven surface, it's uncomfortable but not quite uncomfortable enough to get it to move. So let's start probing for signs of Old Brain thinking with Lite Life challenges:

Lite Life challenges

1　Would your self-image suffer if you lost your job?;
2　Could you bring yourself to move on crisply and cleanly from a difficult emotional relationship?

Still a few Old Brain wrinkles to iron out? Welcome to the human race.

Nothing to lose

It has often been said that the people who fear change most are the ones with the most to lose. Successful middle managers spend much of their time at work protecting their backs. A wealthy rural community may launch a NIMBY ('not in my back yard') campaign against the local government's plans for a new wind farm. Landowners object when walkers are given access to cross their fields.

By contrast, a 20-year-old – and increasingly, a 30-year-old – chucks it all in, and takes a year out to travel the world. And why not? He or she has almost nothing to lose. Neither is tomorrow a problem; for young adults there is so much of it and the horizon of choices is truly vast.

However, the Wisdom of Youth tells us that it is not what we have to lose today that is important. The key consideration is what we will lose tomorrow if we do not change. Stay static and you fall behind. Live a life without change and, very soon, fears and anxieties will crowd in. By failing to change, you sacrifice the future on the altar of the past.

Being flexible is the only way to improve your future. Young Brains have this message encoded in their DNA. It's somewhere deep in yours – you just have to rediscover it.

> 'Only a general who is flexible and knows how to adapt his strategy to changing circumstances can command victorious troops.'
>
> Sun Tzu, *The Art of War*, 500BC

The Lite Life mentality says plan your life *as if* you don't have much to lose. Think about the people you know who are still achieving things in their life. Are these Old Brains holding on to what they've got for dear life? Or are they constantly putting some or all of it at risk? Millionaires, as we know, are frequently ex-bankrupts. The few politicians we trust are held in high esteem because they are prepared to put their reputations on the line by taking up brave new causes. Today's successful careers are built by people who take risks and who learn from failures.

Examples of Lite Life approaches are all around us. In the business world, there is a lot of interest around the ideas of creative destruction and zero-based accounting. Both approaches express the point of view that a good way to create something new is either to destroy what already exists or take a blank sheet of paper and start again

To build success, therefore, business people are being asked to put aside past achievements and start as if they had nothing to lose. This is Young Brain thinking, so why not copy it? What would you do if you lost all your savings? Or if your home was wiped out by a fire?

And yet it is so much easier to stick to the familiar. Even losing a habit or routine can be too tough a decision, too much of a loss. If you find yourself choosing the same dishes in a restaurant or going to the same place on holiday year in year out, then you are part of this syndrome. Holiday homes are part of the constraining baggage of an Old Brain. What about letting it out, and going somewhere different on the income? And while you're in a restaurant, what about choosing an unknown dish or two from the menu? What would you really lose, apart from your Old Brain? Go on. Challenge yourself on some of these smaller things and experience the new you.

Living the Wisdom

Get into the habit of making changes in your life by consciously modifying at least one thing, no matter how small, every single day. Changing the big things will then come more naturally. Practice makes perfect!

The scope for small changes is endless but here are a few for starters. Try an electric toothbrush; walk or cycle to work; add Tabasco to your fried eggs; invite a distant family member to lunch; swap your entire DVD collection with someone else's; visit a different news website; stay up well beyond your normal bedtime to watch a TV programme you don't normally see. You have nothing to lose!

Rejecting roots

Young Brains tend, where possible, to reject attitudes and behaviours which cause their plans to be heavy, slow or irrelevant. The Lite Life approach to planning says: 'Let me be as free and light as possible so that I can react quickly and deftly to take advantage of change.'

For example, in the right circumstances, Young Brains tend towards renting their accommodation rather than buying a flat or house. Why? Quite simply so that they can up sticks when they need to and go where the opportunity presents itself. They don't want to be sitting ducks if the bottom falls out of the local economy, so flexible Young Brains simply move to where it is still booming. Old Brains with deep roots stay put and take their medicine.

Now, we are not suggesting that, if you own a flat or house, you sell up and go on the open road. However, if your circumstances are uncomplicated, you might fancy renting out your home for a while and trying life somewhere different. Notice that this isn't about blithely doing everything the young do, whatever your circumstances, it's about understanding what stale patterns we can fall into, and shaking it up a bit where possible.

This mindset of rejecting roots is again apparent in the job market. Today's Young Brained employees are refusing to commit unconditionally to their career or to their employer. They know that loyalty will often not be reciprocated by employers (witness the downsizing and de-layering processes of many enterprises) and that a job for life is a thing of the past. So they prefer to hang loose, avoid putting down roots and simply plan their next career move. They will go where the next opportunity takes them. The attitudes of so-called 'knowledge workers' is Adaptive Navigation at its best.

An illustration of the lack of commitment of today's employees was given recently by the global human resources director of a huge multinational cosmetics corporation. He'd recently hired a woman who had the perfect CV but who, six months into the job, had not performed to expectations and did not seem fully committed to the job. When questioned, the reason she gave for taking the job in the first place was that it was closest to her home!

To a Young Brain, this makes eminently good sense. Looking at life holistically – rather than through the prism of a life-dominating job – cutting down on commuting is a good move. And, in any case, one job isn't for life so you might as well find a job that fits into your life rather than the other way around.

Seeing these kinds of attitudes, senior managers despair of junior colleagues. But what Old Brains don't understand, is that the freewheeling behaviour of Young Brains is a realistic and often effective response both to a dynamic marketplace and the need to find satisfaction and meaning both within and beyond work.

We see this rejection of roots everywhere we look in society. It extends to: choosing to live life as a single person rather than rushing into marriage; deciding as a couple not to have children; decreasing one's loyalty to brands; and being a swing voter in political elections. In fact any action that takes you out of past practices and away from habits and routines, is a move in favour of a more rootless and reactive Lite Life.

And, like it or not, the roots rejected by Young Brains are often the traditional customs and values espoused by elders. Traditional rules have been listened to and, in some instances, found wanting.

For example, one 'heritage' value concerns 'constancy'. This idea of a stoical response to life's vicissitudes, held dear by Old Brains, is based on the belief that it is important to keep an even temperament whatever the circumstance. This shows discipline over one's emotions and gives others the reassurance that, whatever the situation, they can rely on you and the constancy of your character. The British private school system built the characters of British colonialists upon this very mantra. The stiff-upper-lip approach.

A great example of this form of character-building was witnessed during the battle of Waterloo. In the heat of the conflict, Lord Uxbridge was hit by a shot, turned to the Duke of Wellington and said 'By God, sir. I've lost my leg.' To which Wellington replied 'By God, sir. So you have.'

Young Brains reject this emotionally buttoned-up attitude out of hand. If a situation stimulates them, they get excited. If they are insulted, they get angry. They say that human emotions are, well, human, and to deprive yourself of feelings is to go against the free expression of your personality. Rejecting the obligation to stoicism allows Young Brains to sense the world around them, interact with it on an emotional level and fully engage their passion and enthusiasm in whatever they are doing.

In a world of constant change, the orthodoxy of the past can lose its power and relevance. Certain values and principles are, of course, timeless – fairness, kindness, honesty, looking to help others. But others are less so – constancy, self-control, being right, tradition (for its own sake).

As we said earlier, this means we all need, from time to time, to question the appropriateness of certain values and lifestyles to ensure that they are still relevant.

Maybe you would prefer not to have to ask such difficult questions. Perhaps you would rather live in a world where yesterday is still relevant and where there is a sense of pride to be had in sticking to your guns and staunchly supporting traditional values? Even when you sense in your heart that they are no longer pertinent to some of the questions society asks of us today.

The point is, however, that holding blindly on to the past is becoming more futile than ever. The world is spinning so fast these days, that changing, modifying, mutating and renewing are now the only meaningful approaches that will help us to achieve personal effectiveness.

Living the Wisdom

Give yourself permission to cut yourself free of any family or social obligations, customs and traditions that are holding you back and keeping you rooted in the past.

Completing then creating

Finally, living a Lite Life is about the philosophy of *completing then creating*. Young Brains know that life is complex so they want to keep life as simple and clean as they can. This means moving on. It means rejecting the tyranny of the past and letting go of things.

The obvious example is a broken-down relationship. How many people are devoured by their divorce? Bitterness and recrimination lurk in the very souls of those unable to complete. Change becomes impossible as thoughts continually return to what was done and what was said by the offending ex-partner.

While no one should underestimate the pain and injury felt by someone who has broken off a formerly loving relationship, continually reliving the past is not the way to take on tomorrow's challenges. Stunted in this way, a divorcee places a huge hurdle in the way of finding a new nourishing relationship.

Young Brains suffer from broken relationships too, of course, but have a greater capacity to rebound. And their technique is simple and effective. First complete, then create. This means searching for the way to close a chapter – as a priority. In the case of a relationship, this might be to provoke a divorce. Harsh. Yes. But living a life of misery is no way to prepare for the future with optimism. On a more trivial level, it might mean having an argument with the leader of your group or team in order to clear the air, and to address head-on any issues that are hiding below the surface, in order to get things moving again. It may, more sadly, be about saying goodbye to an old friend who is holding you back.

More prosaically, completing and creating is about doing some of the simple housekeeping tasks well. How many of us are hoarders? We have drawers and cupboards full of useless stuff clogging up our homes. Finally we crack, and decide to do a big spring clean – and send all this junk ... to the garage or attic! Here it stays, mouldering away, for many more years. But you never know, do you? That old biscuit tin might come in handy one day. And who knows when you might next need that infant's carrycot?

Lite Lifers know this to be folly. And so do you. Instinctively, you know that so much junk ties you to the past. Ask yourself this. How did you feel the last time you gritted your teeth and threw away some old encumbrance (a moth-eaten armchair, a stained lampshade, a size 10 pair of flared trousers)? Admit it. You felt liberated and somehow lighter.

This is what we are talking about. Old stuff just nails you to the ground. If you want a feeling of floating freedom, you need to be ruthless with the housekeeping tasks. And the true win-win is when you can help other struggling members of your family, needy friends, your favourite charities or the recycling bin to benefit from all the ballast that you cut away.

Meantime, the vacuum that you create by this spring clean can either be kept minimalist, or filled with items that have more meaning and more relevance to your life today. Remember: complete then create.

In short, leading a Lite Life is a desire to let into your life only what is essential – and the definition of what is essential is anything or anyone who will help you live today and get to the future as a happier, more fulfilled and more effective human being.

Living the Wisdom

Have a big clear-out at home, throwing out all (and we mean *all*) that useless 'stuff' you've been hoarding. Then go out and buy a well-designed signature piece to create a whole new ambience when you come through the front door.

2 Taking 'Street Savvy' decisions

Street Savvy challenges

1 Are you happy making decisions quickly and intuitively, without all of the facts?

2 Do you have a fear of confrontation (and a sneaky feeling the only way you'd hold your own would be to pull rank)?

Young Brains are 'Street Savvy'; that is, they take optimal decisions based on a realistic, real-time assessment of any given situation. A Street Savvy kid is someone who senses danger in the neighbourhood by reading the slightest of clues. Similarly, a Street Savvy Young Brain is rapid, intuitive and smart. The Young Brain naturally looks for streetwise short-cuts to analyse the emerging situation and takes gut-feel decisions based on this snapshot.

The Wisdom of Youth shows us that the patient, structured and logical approach to questions and problems increasingly has limitations in the modern world. The so-called 'scientific methodology' espoused by many an Old Brain has worked pretty well over the years. Today, however, it is often just too time-consuming. In a world where you face tens – even hundreds – of choices every day, decisions need to be taken quickly and intuitively. For instance, faced with the mind-blowing choice of different drink options at Starbucks, emotions trump calculations every time.

From the Young Brain's perspective, rational decision-making is no longer reliable enough to make optimal decisions. Imagine, for instance, that you collect African carvings. You've just found a piece in an antique shop but it's too expensive for your budget. Meanwhile, since it is slightly damaged, you are not completely sure that it is worth the price demanded. Finally, this is a Lega carving which is not the core of your collection. You start mulling over the choice and begin to go around in circles with your logic. So you take pen to paper, divide the page in two and write the pros and cons. A week passes and then another. Do you or don't you? What else could you do with the money? In the end, to your dismay, the carving is bought by someone else while you were dithering. A case of slow thinking and fast regretting.

Logic can tie you up in knots. How do you give weight to price?

To damage? To appropriateness? To feelings of ownership? To the sense of loss if you do lose out to another collector?

The Street Savvy Young Brain looks at this differently. It asks, instinctively, what do I want here? Yes, I confirm I want more African wood sculptures. How do I best go about this? Certainly not by finding one-off examples in my high street antique store. I'd do better to go on eBay, say. Result? The collector finds and buys a perfect Igbo carving, for half the price. No logical check-list is needed. Instinct says that this is a really clever purchase with less risk. No other rationale comes into it.

Living the Wisdom

Next time you have a big decision to make, try this. Rather than just evaluating one course of action versus the other, explore if there is an even better 'third way'; discover the savvier option that lies outside the obvious bipolar choice.

Ready to change

Being Street Savvy means knowing the terrain. While an Old Brain might comfort itself that stability is achievable in life, the Young Brain knows better. It knows that change is the only constant – and therefore readiness for change is the only strategy.

For them, stability is for the birds. The evidence is all around. Middle managers who lose their 'job for life' through downsizing and de-layering; families who lose their 'dream home' due to sub-prime-related foreclosure; married couples whose 'till death us do part' vows end in divorce; employees who find their 'final salary' pension schemes are withdrawn or watered down. Even banks are no longer shown to be immune to change – quite the contrary.

In the public sphere, too, change happens – and happens radically. For example, countries with 'cast iron' welfare state systems are having to make tough choices over funding, and some expensive treatments and drugs are beginning to be withheld. Meanwhile, the recent near bankruptcy of Iceland will not be the last. The IMF (International Monetary Fund) is going to find itself dealing with lots of new challenges over the next few years.

Still believe you can cushion yourself so well that change will not creep into your life? Still feel certain about stability in your corner of the world? Forget it. Americans felt safe at home – until 9/11 and Hurricane Katrina. British farmers felt safe until mad cow disease struck. Even in France, where guaranteed social benefits have been fought for and won over decades, the strength of the guarantee is beginning to dissolve. Kodak felt sure of itself until digital rapidly ruined its marketplace. And say a prayer now for brands such as Wang, Rover, Compaq and Lehman Brothers. Let them rest in peace.

So jobs, homes, marriages, pensions, healthcare and social systems, home security, brands and so on are no longer safe – let alone guaranteed. But, of course, you know all of this. It's just that Young Brains use this knowledge better; their explicit awareness of change ensures that they anticipate change and are always ready to take decisions based on modified circumstances.

Evolution is about changing to survive. Young Brains pick up the signals of how society is changing and respond in ways that enhance their chances of surviving and prospering.

We know a management consultant in his late forties who has been made redundant seven times in his 25-year career. You might have thought, by now, that he would be a broken man and his CV would simply be toxic. Not a bit of it. Today, his earnings are in the top 5 per cent and he is welcomed wherever he goes. A failure? No, merely the product of an unstable world who has a successful strategy to accept change and rebound from setbacks. Indeed, he has integrated change to such an extent that, today, the first thing he does when joining a company is to negotiate his redundancy terms! Being laid off can be profitable and liberating.

Young Brains are excellent bell-wethers concerning change and watching them closely will help you to react to how the world is evolving. Even better, is developing *your* ability to detect social dynamics and adapt to trends.

Perhaps you grew up being told not to question things. To take things at face value. Now's the chance to reject all of that. Most things can be altered; there is little that is really fixed in today's world.

Living the Wisdom

Make a list of seven disasters that potentially could hit your life and plan how you would rebound from each. Use a 'Street Savvy' approach to finding 'third way' solutions rather than usual linear thinking. For example, an unfortunate long-term illness might give you just the chance you need to fulfil your ambition to learn Spanish.

Trial-and-error learning

It is one thing being ready to make changes but it is quite another to make decisions. Whereas Old Brains are methodical about accumulating facts and figures, making lists of pros and cons and finally thinking things through logically, Young Brains have a radically different approach as we saw above. In many cases, they take decisions through a trial-and-error approach.

A simple way to illustrate the difference between the old and Young Brain methods is to take the example of a newly arrived plasma-screen TV. The Old Brain, happy that his purchase has finally arrived, opens the box carefully and removes the instruction manual. This, incidentally, runs to 480 pages, but that's okay as only 60 of these are in English. The Old Brain proceeds by reading this 'book' from the starting 'Safety Instructions' right through to 'How to Assemble the Stand Base' at the back. Confident that all the information has been read and absorbed, the Old Brain now, and only now, dares to extract the TV from its polystyrene protection and plug it into the wall (with only a passing glance, now, at the instructions to reread the 'Switching Your Television On and Off' section).

Enter the Young Brain. Step one: rip the box asunder. Step two: plug in. Step three: try to watch. Step four: sort out the lack of picture by 'playing' with the remote control a bit. Step five: watch.

From here on in it's plain sailing for the Young Brain, as any further problems are resolved by repeating step four.

You've watched teenagers using computers or mobile phones. They have no fear or worry. They 'navigate' the menus and instructions, often only half pausing to read what's written before clicking and clicking again. And, hey presto, it's done. An Old Brain (and don't worry, the authors are with you on this one) gets to a drop-down menu with items that mean nothing, panics, and tries to find their way back to safer ground.

The terror for the Old Brain is where your computer asks you if you want to download the update. Will this seemingly wise thing to do completely mess up your PC's configuration? Will the teetering tower of patches and partial updates come crashing down following a momentary madness when you accepted this new software?

With the Young Brains' mindset, such technophobia is incomprehensible. You don't need to know everything to take decisions, you don't even need to be in partial control of the facts. You just need a spirit of adventure, and a trial and error approach to get you through. And if you cock up, continue trialling and erroring until you get it sorted.

Interestingly, many technological companies are now applying this approach to assessing their new products. Rather than lab testing everything before deciding to launch, they send out a beta version and see what comments come back. And the reason they do this? They get better, quicker answers by using customers as co-inventors. Customers know how they will use the devices, and can often see new applications that conventional analysis would never have arrived at. The millions of text messages sent every day would not have been possible if customers had not taken SMS technology and used it in ways that the developers' analytical approach had never envisaged.

The reason this may lead to better decisions and outcomes is that a more comprehensive and creative exploration of the alternatives in this process of iteration often produces results that would have been unlikely through traditional methods of analysis. In the same way that solutions from other industries often transform traditional markets (would the makers of car maps have come up with satnavs?), so a wider scoping of ideas can often produce a better answer than could have been arrived at by analysis, however careful and painstaking.

It is significant that one of the reasons that trial-and-error learning has become popular relates to how other forms of learning have declined – in particular learning through 'transmission'.

Transmission is the process whereby society passes on past learning to future generations. Transmission can be about what is right or wrong, good or bad – but it's also about the practical things in life: how to cook; how to mend things; and how to study and learn. When a father shows his son or daughter how to rewire a plug, that's transmission.

From the very earliest tribal societies with their oral tradition, transmission has worked more or less effectively – until recently, that is.

From about the late 1960s (no coincidence that this corresponds to the student and hippie movements around the world), transmission began breaking down in many Western societies. The evidence? Simple. You only have to look at the abundance of 'how to' lifestyle programmes on television today to realise that there is a huge gap in many people's learning that TV now fills. Younger generations now learn more from outside sources than from their parents when it comes to cooking, repairing, gardening or even child-rearing.

And here's the point. In the context of low levels of transmission, Young Brains have got used to finding their own trial-and-error ways to cope with the daily challenges of life – as opposed to turning to traditional ways and heritage solutions.

You don't know how to cook a traditional meal? No problem, the high street takeaway offers fast food from five continents, or you can bung a few things in a pan and see how it turns out. You're not sure about parenting? Not to worry, as Doctor Spock tells to-be parents: 'You already know more than you think.'

Translated, he is saying: 'Just do it, muddle through and proceed by trial and error. You'll get there.'

> You can discover a great deal about how society is changing by noting what comedians poke fun at. In the 1990s there was a British comedy show filled with a cast of characters acted by Harry Enfield. One particularly annoying character was a dad who repeated parrot-fashion to his son: 'You don't want to do it like that; you want to do it like this.' The crux of the humour was how ridiculous parents are when they try to transmit their learning to a younger generation. A sure sign that society was turning against traditional parental wisdom and teaching, and moving towards a more instinctive, self-taught, trial-and-error approach to decision-making.

Living the Wisdom

Next time you buy a new electrical or electronic device, look at the safety instructions and then cast the manual aside. Play, navigate, explore. And continue experimenting over time to find more and more functionality.

Decide real quick

Young Brains like to make decisions quickly. Of course, if you are ready for change and are prepared to proceed by trial and error, instantaneous decisions become possible – even desirable.

Life is accelerating and pace gives you natural advantage. Concert tickets are put on sale at 08h30. Only the first comers are served. The boat excursion to the island is in two days' time. The early birds get the remaining places. The school ski trip has limited numbers. Only boys and girls with reactive parents get to go.

Today, dithering and procrastination stifle life-chances like never before. Without the capacity to decide rapidly, you will miss the concert, be stuck at the back of the boat and have your kids not speak to you for a week.

Americans say that you have to make decisions 'real quick' – and they are right. Street Savvy Young Brains recognise the need to be spontaneous – and they reap the rewards of this fast flexibility. It's all about being quick and clever, rather than ponderous and considered. It's Young Brain wisdom.

For example, when Young Brains go shopping they adaptively navigate the store. While Old Brains have shopping lists, Young Brain shoppers decide impulsively according to what's on offer. Accordingly, the rates of spontaneous purchases have risen sharply over recent years. A recent Harris Poll survey found that 50 per cent of British grocery shoppers did not forward plan their shopping. They reacted rapidly to what they saw on the shelves, rather than working from a shopping list. This is Street Savvy at work.

Talking of supermarkets, did you imagine that the special offer displays at your local supermarket were just for the price-conscious? Think again. Young Brains use these bargain bins to blend a basket of untried, unknown items. Then, once home, they will adapt to their basket's contents and rustle up some sort of spontaneous fusion meal. Not for them recipe books. It's more, a pinch of intuition, a dash of inspiration and a good dose of luck. Hey presto, a meal cooked from items on promotion – and probably then eaten by a fairly spontaneous gathering of friends that just happened to drop by.

Incidentally, this example neatly illustrates neatly how far the Street Savvy strategy can permeate many aspects of life: from purchasing patterns, to cooking and eating habits, to handling personal relationships.

There is a TV programme called *Ready, Steady, Cook* which you might have seen. In it, recognised chefs are paired up with members of the public who bring along a mystery bag of groceries. The chefs have just 20 minutes to concoct a meal with the ingredients. Without fail, our Young Brained chefs turn the surprise ingredients into a magic mouth-watering meal. Could you?

Living the Wisdom

Break the mould by spontaneously buying foods you normally pass over at the supermarket (pigs' trotters, green bananas, kumquats – you get the idea). Spend the week preparing and eating experimental dishes.

This particular navigation could have the additional benefit of helping you be thrifty, when financial times are tough. Being open to change allows you to flex your spending and cut your cloth according to swings in your income.

Complaining and exiting

When we talk of Adaptive Navigation, we also talk about the ability to change course if where you are heading is not where you want to be. The Street Savvy attitude is about just this. Put crudely, someone who is Street Savvy knows when to pull the plug.

As we work through what it means to be Young Brained, it would be easy to come to the conclusion that they are always taking the easy option or the path of least resistance. Look at what we have said already. By not putting down roots, you could argue that Young Brains lack commitment. And by not doing the legwork required to buff up on the facts and figures, they take 'lazy' instinctive decisions. However, in neither case are these easy options. Simple, yes – easy, no. Living a Lite Life can be emotionally testing. And taking spontaneous decisions requires courage. Likewise, when it comes to pulling the plug, this is often the most difficult of all options.

We have said that to be Street Savvy requires you to know the terrain – and specifically when it comes to complaining and exiting, this means knowing exactly what your rights and responsibilities are. It is no good complaining about a late home delivery if you failed to communicate when you'd be available.

Young Brains are awake to what they can expect and by the same token, what they need to do.

For example, they know that when entering a restaurant they must be respectful of others. They also expect a certain level of reciprocated respect, high-quality service and appropriate ambience. If this equation does not add up, being Young Brained means being able to explain your grievance, get up, walk out and go somewhere else.

However, if you are Old Brained and not open to making rapid decisions based on your emotions, chances are that you feel a social pressure to stay put. And, by the way, muttering your dissatisfaction under your breath doesn't cut it. So, if you've sat still in an appalling restaurant quietly fuming and telling yourself you'll never return, be prepared in the future to challenge that Old Brained thinking. Assert your rights and exit. And remember that you are not only helping to improve service levels for those diners after you, but, more importantly, you are striking a blow against your own mental inertia. You moved on. Pat yourself on the back.

Note that the exiting bit is important. There is nothing an Old Brain likes better than complaining. But, without exiting, it's not being Street Savvy. So next time you're in a store and the service is poor, make sure you make your point and then leave, rather than grumbling after you've paid for the goods.

Another aspect of complaining and exiting relates to the fact that most things nowadays are seen to be negotiable. The price tag on that sofa? Negotiable. The restaurant bill after a disappointing meal? The coffee should be offered free of charge. The second-class airline ticket. An upgrade is possible. All that is required is the courage to provoke change. The change in perception that comes from saying that you really cannot afford the price being charged, that you are a dissatisfied customer, that you know that they have the power and space to upgrade you.

Living the Wisdom

It's happened to all of us – we need a workman to fix something at home and the result we get is shoddy and/or overpriced. Next time this happens to you, complain until you get satisfaction. Afterwards, feel proud that you've been 'Street Savvy'.

In short, Street Savvy means being ready to change, learning through trial and error, making quick decisions, and being prepared to complain and/or exit when you find you are heading in the wrong direction. As an approach to decision-making, it is less about facts and more about feelings; less about analysing, more about doing; less about the fear of failure and more about the fun of finding.

For a Young Brain, if you want to do something in your life, have a little think about alternatives, listen to what your gut is saying and then dive in – adjusting as you go. Analysis takes place on the run, and readjustment and improvement are real-time dynamics. This is Street Savvy decision-making at work – and it's an approach that is open to anyone and everyone who wants to rejuvenate.

3 Gender Blending

Gender Blending challenges

1 Do you tend to decide what you will do and the roles you are prepared to play on the basis of your gender?

2 Are you comfortable with the fact that women are gaining more power and influence in the world?

As we said earlier, Adaptive Navigation also comes down to negotiating who does what. The Young Brained answer is: whatever works; and whatever is most appropriate in the circumstances. The Old Brained approach is: whatever is traditional and linked to old-fashioned hierarchical rules of social standing.

There are many relationships where Young Brains look to recast the responsibility for who does what. Parents and their children. Bosses and employees. Committees and workers. Governments and voters. In this section, we've chosen to illustrate how just one set of relationships gets mediated by Young Brains i.e. how the sexes relate.

Modern life asks fairly fundamental questions about human relationships and particularly about gender roles. Gender Blending describes a relevant new way of seeing the relationship between the sexes and it embodies the Adaptive Navigation mindset.

Young Brains are extremely impatient with conventional wisdom – if conventional wisdom has no merit. And traditional gender roles are exactly that – conventional wisdom with no merit. The concept whereby 'the woman always stays at home looking after the kids and the man is always the breadwinner' simply does not compute in the Young Brain's head.

For a Young Brain, this concept of gender roles is an Old Brained posture – a throwback to a historically male-dominated society. Today, life's challenges are such that Young Brains understand that the only wise way to react is by using the talents of everybody – whatever their gender. So forget tradition and macho ways.

This again is reasoning that comes hard to some Old Brainers. Whatever the achievements of women's liberation, there are still generations of men out there fighting hard to deny equal opportunities, turning a blind eye to women's talents. Some men are fighting a rearguard action to keep glass ceilings firmly in place (while, of course, pretending not to). It's like the celebrated case of the Japanese soldier, Hiroo Onada, found on an isolated island 29 years after the Second World War had ended, who was still fighting the war. Old Brains are still fighting the battle of the sexes, long after younger generations have accepted and welcomed Gender Blending.

Living the Wisdom

Rethink roles and talents at your workplace or within a club or association to which you belong. Could there be a more sensible and beneficial way of allocating the tasks that need doing? For example, why is Harry repairing the gutter when he's great at arranging flowers? Why is Marge making the coffee when her persuasive skills could be deployed convincing a major donor to give even more?

Horses for courses

While we have some way to go to arrive at equality between men and women, both in the developed as well as the developing world, Gender Blending recognises the simple truth that it makes sense for men and women to vary their roles at different moments in time.

The Young Brain approach is for a couple to negotiate, on an ongoing basis, who does what and when. It might be that, during the week, the woman keeps the kids and the man goes out to work. At weekends, the man is childminding while the woman works with the charity she supports. The woman may abandon her high-flying career during child-rearing years, but it's the husband who takes over the domestic responsibilities when the woman's small business takes off.

An important part of this, of course, is common sense and convenience. But for Young Brains it's important to note that personal development comes into it too. For many couples, living a life of fulfilment and meaning is important, so space has to be freed up to achieve this. Both partners will therefore play a part in the allocation of roles to make it happen.

The point is, change happens and it's in both partners' interests to find flexible and fair responses to new situations. Such a balanced way of perceiving gender roles helps enormously and gives greater security to the couple. The man's new job is closer to the school? Great, then he picks up the kids. The woman's career is going great guns – then her job takes priority.

Contrast this with Old Brain thinking. In the UK, the coal and steel communities in the early 1980s had serious confrontations with the government of Margaret Thatcher. The miners and steelworkers – virtually all men – were laid off in swathes and became hugely despondent because they were no longer the breadwinners. Tradition said that it was the man's role to work and the woman's to raise the children. How many households could have rebounded with greater speed, if an early decision had been taken to reverse the roles in the household?

Living the Wisdom

Sit down with your partner (if you have one) and list the tasks and roles involved in daily life. Then freshly and clinically reappraise the existing allocation according to the talent and time available. Find at least one area of life where role reversal is entirely appropriate and make the switch.

Women on top

The need for Gender Blending becomes much more obvious when we acknowledge how far society has become feminised and how much women have to offer a fully functioning and globalised world.

For example, while Gender Blending is more advanced in the Western world, it is significant that, when you look at global developments, the biggest changes to existing social value systems are being provoked by women.

From Japan to Jakarta and from Spain to Saudi Arabia, the influence of women on social values is being felt on two fronts. The first is the battle to be recognised as equal to men. The second is the spread of 'feminine' values (such as intuition, emotion and empathy), which are pushing societies in new feminised directions.

Meanwhile, although some Old Brain men still resist it, women, by and large, are becoming as well equipped, arguably better equipped, to be the leaders in many areas of life, especially the workplace.

There are several reasons for this. Firstly, in many countries, women are simply better educated today. There are more girls in higher education than boys and they get better exam results. Secondly, they are, by and large, more intuitive than men, and, therefore better suited to Adaptive Navigation. Thirdly, they are better at multitasking – a talent increasingly in demand as life becomes more complicated and pressurised.

Finally, women tend to be at better interpersonal skills. They have more empathy, are more interested in, and understanding of, other people. They have higher emotional intelligence (EI) and relate more naturally to their fellow human beings, and care more about them. In the flat hierarchies emerging in most organisations in the developed world, interpersonal skills are probably the most important of all skills in achieving effectiveness and success.

So, with the percentage of manual jobs reducing to very low levels in developed societies, women are at least as well qualified, and possibly more qualified, to became the major household income earner. In fact, this is already the case in 55 per cent of US households, where women bring in more than half of the income. And while American men's median incomes rose by 0.6 per cent in the years between 1970 and 1998, women's median income rose by some 63 per cent (quoted in Tom Peters, *Essentials: Trends*).

These statements and these facts are, of course, profoundly uncomfortable for Old Brains and male Old Brains in particular.

But, appreciating these new realities is the first step in moving away from old discriminatory habits and thoughts.

And if all this sounds too stereotypical, we apologise. Some people have blended genders already and this will be very familiar to them. Young Brains may be doing it as a matter of course, but older brains are not. If you are one of these, try very hard to get with it. Understand that blurring gender roles has nothing to do with your sexual orientation but may have everything to do with how adaptable you are to the massive changes in the daily world around you.

Living the Wisdom

Choose at least one woman you respect and learn from her as a role model. Choose at least one woman as a sporting hero and a music idol respectively. Tell the world of the admiration you have for these women whenever appropriate. Better still, actively seek to have a talented female boss.

By the way, these recommendations apply whether you are male or female.

As we have said, this chapter is the big one. Rediscover your ability to accept and adapt to change and you will be able to navigate through life – and, most importantly, make progress with the other five wisdoms we now move on to.

SUMMARY OF GOALS

- Clarify your basic principles which you will not compromise; be ready to realign and update other values in keeping with contemporary society.

- Give up your comfort zones one by one.

- Challenge your habits, rituals and routines; force yourself to unlock the shackles holding you down; live a Lite Life.

- Take Street Savvy decisions – intuitively and quickly.

- Reprioritise and blend tasks with your partner.

04

Enlightened Selfishness

'I did it! I did it!' Claire hugged herself with joy.

She felt great. About herself, and the situation. The nursery she worked in at last recognised how good she was with the children, and how the parents valued her. Not only had she got an increase in pay, she would now only be working the statutory hours – no unpaid overtime. And she even had a new man in her life.

Was it only six months ago she had resolved to stop being used by everyone? The kindergarten had been dumping all the difficult kids on her. And the parents had been late picking them up, knowing she wouldn't complain.

Her self-regard had been low, she'd been overweight, and things were getting worse. Then she'd found an article in a magazine on building self-confidence and finding fulfilment. She'd followed what it recommended. She'd exercised regularly, read self-development books and got out socially, meeting more people.

Finally, today, she'd confronted her employers at the playgroup. The two managers had been taken aback. They'd gone away and talked about it, and had come back and agreed to all her demands. There seemed to be a new respect in their eyes.

Yes. She'd done it.

Defining Enlightened Selfishness

It's a sad fact but many of us, like the 'old' Claire, tend to get lost in our own lives. We lose direction and shape. All those heady youthful ambitions, all that clarity of what you wanted to achieve in life can somehow get muddled and mislaid. Suddenly, we wake to the feeling that we count for much less than we supposed. We amount to less that we'd hoped for. Meanwhile, the drive has gone, along with the spark; others are running past us and we are just dragging our heels.

Of course, we all come up with quite reasonable alibis to justify falling short of our expectations from youth. We had a bad accident and never quite recovered. Someone close passed away and this hit us badly. The shock of redundancy knocked us for six. But, despite our endless resourcefulness at justification and post-rationalisation, in the dead of a sleepless night, when truth prevails, we look into our hearts and admit our own failings. Often, we finally understand that we lost the plot because we simply failed to look out for our own best interests.

Ever felt like this? Ever wondered how you ended up being everyone else's dogsbody? Ever questioned where things went wrong? Exactly at what part of your life did you lose vision and start living day to day; wandering aimlessly through life? Or when the precise moment was that you stopped respecting yourself, sticking up for yourself, improving yourself?

No one lives an entirely charmed life and we all have setbacks – even the rich and successful. But Young Brains know that it is important to protect yourself from life's knocks by, first and foremost, looking after your own needs. Failure to do so means that not only are you far less able to attend to the needs of others around you but the consequences on your own sense of self-worth can be devastating and long-lasting.

Enlightened selfishness, then, is all about developing and retaining your self-esteem which, as the wisdom suggests, often requires putting your needs above all others – at least temporarily. It means listening to yourself, investing in yourself and making your own requirements explicit to others. By doing yourself this favour, you avoid frustration and sidestep destructive self-criticism.

And here's the important point. By focusing first on your own needs and development, you then liberate yourself to do good for others. Indeed, you become better at helping others because you do so from a position of self-respect and personal strength. This is the 'enlightened' bit.

So we are not recommending that you become completely selfish. Not in the least. We are saying that you need to avoid both the extremes of pure selfishness and pure giving.

Developing yourself

'People don't grow old. When they stop growing, they become old.'

Anon.

The Wisdom of Youth is that we are more effective if other people find us attractive. Not just physically, but as human beings they want to be near and with. Many young people are naturally attractive and very conscious of their attractiveness. They use it in positive ways to get things done and make things happen. They are self-confident, energetic and enthusiastic. They have plans, visions and lots of self-esteem. Their boldness has magic in it. Enlightened selfishness is all about rediscovering your personal magic.

I would like to develop different aspects of my personality more fully in my everyday life

	15–17	18–24	25–34	35–44	45–54	55–64	65+
% Agree	80	81	78	75	69	65	43

Source: Sociovision 3SC UK, 2005

Young people are more naturally inclined to keep on the self-development trail. But from the age of 25 our desire to improve ourselves wanes. Again, we start to abandon our ambitions very early in our lives. Older generations truly get lost in their own lives and, from 65 onwards, the majority believe that it's all done and dusted.

This Wisdom of Youth is a recognition that developing yourself and your personality is vital. Moreover, it is an ongoing process and not something to be left behind along with your teenage years.

It is worth acknowledging, before we go any further, that 'self-help' and 'personal development' have had a somewhat alternative image over the years – particularly in certain cultures. It has been mocked by the ignorant. 'After all,' they say, 'who but the socially stunted would read books with titles such as *How to Win Friends and Influence People*'?

In fact, Dale Carnegie's book is a classic and, with justification, still sells massively. It is a brilliant exposition of some core life skills. Winning friends and influencing people sounds manipulative (he probably wouldn't have used that title if he were publishing it today) but its core message is central to effective living: in families, in work and in social life. It is 70 years since he wrote it, and it is still fresh and relevant today.

Personal development is, in essence, developing your life skills so you can be more effective at helping yourself and others to live a more worthwhile, enjoyable and fulfilling life. It is about being stimulated by, and engaged in, life.

Part of this, of course, is freeing yourself from the anxieties (those curses of the Old Brain) of not being able to cope – with work, life or being a human being. The more knowledge and insight you have into the best ways to survive and thrive, the more chance you will have of enjoying life. We all have setbacks, and failures. We all have feelings that we are losing the plot. Personal development in all its forms – coaching, books, courses, workshops, electronic media, and general ideas and knowledge-sharing – help us to grow as individuals and arm us with the experience and insights of others into the best way of making a decent fist of it.

It is rightly said that 'Leaders are readers'. Leaders are constantly expanding their knowledge base. You need knowledge to be a leader of your own biography. No information – no insights. No insights – no progress and no innovation.

So, personal development is crucial to staying Young Brained. Only Old Brains knock it.

Benefits of developing enlightened selfishness

A lifetime of learning and self-advancement has many benefits.

- Gaining insight and energy from personal development.
- Becoming an interesting person whom others want to spend time with.
- Loving more (from a solid base where you love and respect yourself).
- Living rich, interdependent relationships with others (and thus avoiding the pitfalls of dependence or independence).
- Being more open emotionally.
- Getting full satisfaction from your volunteering (rather than minimising it under the dead hand of duty).
- Feeling healthier, looking better and performing optimally.
- Standing up for yourself.
- Focusing your actions on your sphere of influence (thus avoiding the distractions of things you cannot affect).

Self talk

As you work on your own personal rejuvenation, we hope you'll come back to this book time and again to guide and encourage you. But there is another support that you'll be able to tap into to guide your transition, and that is your younger self. Remember we said that most of us lost the Wisdom of Youth en route and much of this book is about rediscovering what you already know. It should be obvious, then, that somewhere deep inside your subconscious are Young Brain thought patterns. It's just that they got forgotten, left behind and replaced by older brain thoughts as time went by.

What if you could recall these submerged thoughts to accelerate your progress towards a younger you?

The great news is that you can! And the technique to access these, we call 'self-talk'. Yes, that's right. We want you to talk to yourself. Not out loud maybe, but who's to stop you if that's how you want to do it? More likely, though, it will be an inner voice in your head.

What does this voice say? Basically, it is a supportive, encouraging, daring voice that tells you to get on and change values, challenge comfort zones and radically change mindsets. And it is a voice that pushes you to make changes to your behaviour; it stimulates you into 'Living the Wisdom'.

It works like this. As we have started to do in Chapter 3, and we'll continue to do in this chapter and beyond, we'll give you the insights and things to do to rejuvenate your mind and so raise your YQ. We want you to reawaken your Young Brain and allow it, initially, to coexist with your older brain. *The voice inside doing the self-talk should be your Young Brain.*

Let's give an example to offset any understandable scepticism you may have. Later in this chapter we'll be recommending that you (re)read some of the self-development classics. You initial reaction may be to resist and find lots of 'legitimate' reasons why you couldn't possibly take this advice. This is your dominant older brain talking. So here's the chance to awaken your Young Brain and do some convincing self-talk. Let your mind remember how it used to enjoy gaining new knowledge, how excited you became when exploring a new subject that interested you, how brilliant you felt when telling people what you'd learned.

Some readers will find this easy, while others may have to dig back to, say, infant school to resurrect memories of their enthusiastic learning.

Next, allow your Young Brain to talk you into new thoughts and actions. So you say to yourself: 'I should really read those books, they'll be interesting, get me excited, give me something to say at work or over coffee. I must get hold of them, before the end of the week and read one each fortnight. Yes, that's what I'll do and I'll feel really good about myself when I've done it. I am on my way to a younger mindset.'

Of course, as the months go by, your goal should be that the Young Brain voice becomes increasingly persuasive and eventually so dominant that it almost entirely replaces your older brain's tired discourse. When you have reach this point, you can reduce the *conscious* Young Brain self-talk, because it will now be the *unconscious* whole. You will be young again!

A final word, we've introduced 'self-talk' here because it falls so neatly within the topic of enlightened selfishness. It is a method that will help you work on yourself. However, it should be obvious that it is absolutely relevant to support any and every wisdom.

Let's return to this wisdom and look at which mindsets you'll be needing to talk yourself into.

Adopt three enlightened selfishness mindsets as your own

Personal development is an important part of this wisdom, but it is not the whole story. It is a challenging wisdom in several ways and, once more, it will cause you to challenge certain values you may have grown up with and hold dear. For example, you may need to square what we are saying here with the edict to 'serve others', if that is deeply embedded in your DNA. Or another example of how you could find your values challenged. If you are a devoted young parent, it can be heart-wrenching to put time aside for your own needs when you have little ones clamouring for your attention. We will discuss this later in the chapter.

And again, we will be challenging you out of your comfort zones. For example, you might have got quite comfortable with the idea that you'll never have to do another arduous physical workout in your life. Perhaps you believed you had left that behind at school along with the gymslips and the pommel horse? Again, we will be shaking some of these easy-life notions as we go through.

But the payback comes when you start to adopt the lessons of this wisdom comprehensively; when you start to re-programme your old or Middle-aged Brain with three Young Brain mindsets:

- Acknowledging Your Power
- Generating Self-esteem
- Helping Others

1 Acknowledging your power

Power challenges

1 How far do you consider that, on your own, you can influence the political debate?

2 If you see a big corporate doing something you dislike, do you believe you can change things?

You are in the pilot's seat

Young Brains are a bit like canaries down mines. They give an early warning of an alteration in the atmosphere. They are the first to sense the winds of change and move on. Older brains would do well to watch them and react accordingly.

Watching how Young Brains think and behave today tells us that more and more that we live in a 'bottom-up' society where power is in the hands of the individual.

For example, when a Young Brain has a political grievance, she will not wait until election time but will launch a blog to air her views and gain wider acceptance of her opinions. Can this be influential? You bet! It is interesting to note how far the 2008 Democratic nominee campaign in the US was driven by Web-based donations, opinions, questions and campaign management.

Obama's supporters were net natives. They knew how to use the medium to spread their messages. 'Obama owes his victory to the internet. He used the web more effectively than any prior national candidate, harnessing its organizing power to vault over ... Hillary Clinton ... with an enormous internet-driven donor base of 1.5 million people, more than 800,000 of whom have accounts on Obama's social networking website ... his online supporters have created more than 30,000 events to promote his candidacy.'   Wired.com

Suddenly, the election was less about the party machine, and more about 30,000 supporters getting engagement and money at a grassroots level. Obama captured this new power of the individual to help him over the line. Politics will never be seen in the same way again.

Outside of politics, other Young Brains willingly pass on the benefits of their experiences of products and services to fellow Young Brains through a multitude of evaluation websites. Tripadvisor.com gives reviews of holidays and hotels; Askanowner.com solicits replies from current product users; and, of course, Amazon.com allows readers to post their own appreciation of the book they read. In fact, there is a ratings site for almost everything. Shopping: epinions.com; restaurants: dinesite.com; technology: geek.com. And so it goes on.

The point to note here is that an individual's review or comment sometimes has the power to make or break whatever is being evaluated. The power of word of mouth could always make or break brands and products, but it frequently took a long, long time. The web has massively accelerated this power and made it lethal.

A 50-year-old lock design was rendered useless in 2004 when a brief post to an Internet forum revealed the lock could be popped open with a cheap plastic pen. The brand was forced to launch a lock exchange offer. In another Youtube video, a combination lock is opened with no tools in less than 30 seconds. Both brands' businesses were severely jeopardised almost overnight as a consequence of these postings by individuals.

Examples also abound of the power of individuals to group together in an informal, organic way and put pressure on the big boys.

www.tescopoly.org was, quote: 'launched in June 2005 to highlight and challenge the negative impacts of Tesco's [the UK's biggest supermarket] behaviour along its supply chains both in the UK and internationally, on small businesses, on communities and the environment. The campaign also advocates national and international legislation needed to curb the market power of all the major British supermarkets.'

Result: in 2006, Tesco responded by putting a Community Plan at the heart of its brand values. Chief Executive Sir Terry Leahy stated: 'The message from our customers is that they want to be empowered to make more sustainable choices and they want to see Tesco active in their community.'

The message is clear. Informal groupings of individuals now have the power to create policy, even within the biggest of corporations. It is increasingly the grass-roots that influence how things progress, not the big boots at the top.

What has this got to do with enlightened selfishness? Everything. Because, in a world where politicians, big business, big institutions, etc. are ceding power to the individual, it means that you have take more responsibility for your life. Increasingly, it's *you* in the pilot's seat.

Moreover, it is up to you and me to control our own lives and outcomes because no-one else is doing it for us any more. In today's economy, we are all being charged to take responsibility for more aspects of our lives as the state and employers reduce their roles.

So, all of us, individually, have to step up to the plate. If no-one else is in control, each of us has to control our own lives. This Wisdom has been integrated by Young Brains. This is why they put faith in enlightened selfishness.

Young Brains carve out some time to develop themselves and

their capacities because they know that, quite simply, they have to take on more and more responsibility. This is not the moment in history to be deferential or to sit back content with what you have already learned. The onus is on each and every one of us to be in the pilot's seat. We need to train ourselves to be able to fly.

Living the Wisdom

If you want to flex your political muscle, one of the most useful actions you can take over the next few weeks and months is to understanding and begin using online pressure groups. Spend some time just exploring websites that tackle your particular bugbear and start joining the debate forums. The bigger goal is to set up a blog of your own which becomes both popular and influential. If you use www.blogger.com, this is both easy and free!

2 Generating Self-esteem

Self-respect challenges

1 When did you last create 'ME' time to devote to your own needs or to invest in your own interests?
2 Are you taking regular exercise and do you feel good about your body?

Virtually everyone suffers from a lack of self-esteem, from time to time. Even the most optimistic people sometimes question their own abilities and sense of worth. Does this surprise you? It shouldn't. After all, we are all human.

For example, anyone turning to drugs or engaging in self-harm is revealing themselves to be lacking in self-respect. How many people like that do you know? Hollywood stars, too, are renowned for going from incredible highs to almost bottomless lows, as their celebrity status waxes and wanes and deepest doubts creep in.

Knowing that it's only human to have self-doubts and be self-critical does not make it any easier to live with, though, does it? If you have low self-esteem, most things begin to seem like an insurmountable challenge; most contacts with others start to feel embarrassing – even threatening. The problem with being down on yourself is that it saps your energy and disempowers you.

The wisdom of enlightened selfishness tells us that self-esteem is something of such high value – and such an important foundation for so many other good things in life – that it must be consciously cultivated at all times. And that means that *you* need to be actively looking after it; no one else is going to do it. In other words, in this aspect of life, you have to be entirely selfish.

And, of course, it's absolutely worth it. Ask yourself the question: Would I rather go through life with my head held high, bringing my unique contribution to bear, or am I happy living in the shadows, unhappy often, even to show my face?

Living the Wisdom

Get out of any negativity spiral by forming a more realistic assessment of who you are and what you bring to the world. Chances are you underestimate your positives, so do this exercise. Title three pieces of paper, respectively: Past successes; My skills and strengths; and Why others like me. Systematically fill each page by drawing upon examples taken from daily life – today and in the past. Stand back and absorb the fact that, really, you are not so bad after all. Are you?

Inner development

This is a key aim of the Young Brain. It is where personal development comes into its own. If we are wise, we all continue to learn about the world around us, stretch our minds and stimulate our intellects. The Wisdom of Youth puts this into practice. Young Brains are brains that never stop discovering. Curiosity about countries, a passion about peoples, science, local history, philosophy – you name it. Geeks used to be mocked; now they are (almost) cool.

A lifetime of learning means always having a book by your bedside. It means travelling far and wide. It's about being open to change – as we've already said. It means getting yourself enrolled on the adult education class in needlework, Portuguese or computing. It means taking that weekend cookery class – or attending seminars at a figurative painting school. It can also mean learning more about child-rearing from TV's *Supernanny*!

Whatever you do, however you do it, self-development is important. Not only to keep yourself stimulated and alive – although that's positive and desirable. But also to feed your sense of self-esteem. You are aiming to be the best you can be. You are getting to like and love yourself. Yes, you are also being selfish. However, the greater goal is that you become a more loving, lovable and interesting person as a result.

Steven Covey's best-seller *The Seven Habits of Highly Effective People* talks about the private victories that must come before public victories. He argues cogently that 'the decision to be the creative force of our own lives is the most fundamental choice of all. It is the heart and soul of being a transition person. It is the essence of becoming an agent of change.'

In essence, it's about developing your integrity. How can you be honest with others if you cannot be honest with yourself? Will you really be able to prove it to others, if you haven't first proven it to yourself? Look at it another way: will others respect you if they see what a downer you have on yourself and your own individuality? Here's how educator David O. McKay put it: 'the greatest battles of life are fought out daily in the silent chambers of the soul.' If you want to do good to others, first do good to yourself. That's how Young Brains think.

Former Arsenal and England football captain Tony Adams went through a long sequence of alcohol-related embarrassments which he details honestly in his book *Addicted*. When he finally asked for help he says that his 29-year-old's athlete's body had felt more like a 60-year-old man's. Coming out of the tunnel, he set up the Sporting Chance Clinic in 2000, as a charity to help alcoholic sports people, and also went back to Brunel University to study 'the social anthropology of football'. Here was a famous man who had hit the wall by the time he was 30 but who then invested in his own development, and was able to find constructive new outlets to help others through similar difficulties.

It's worth adding, too, that all this self-development work can only but help you socially. For example, it's a bit of a misnomer to talk about 'self-help' books because, very often, you'll find, they are as much about improving interpersonal relationships and social skills as they are about purely personal development. For this reason alone, they are a must.

Living the Wisdom

Have a personal development book or course on the go. Put aside any scepticism of self-help literature, get your inner voice going and plunge into the classics. For example: Susan Jeffers' *Feel the Fear and do it anyway*; Dale Carnegie's *How to Win Friends and Influence People*; David Schwartz's *The Magic of Thinking Big*; Steven Covey's *The Seven Habits of Highly Effective People*.

Body culture

Enlightened selfishness is also a result of work on your physical well-being.

Here's a couple of impertinent questions for you. How sexy are you? How charismatically appealing are you? Maybe you can answer these questions very positively and, if so, congratulations. But if you hesitated, blushed, refused to treat the questions seriously or answered negatively, then you need more Young Brain wisdom in your life.

You can never be too old to escape from needing attractiveness, even sex appeal. You are never freed from the physical impression you create. Older brains might think that one of the benefits of being aged is that they no longer need to play such 'superficial games'. This is, unfortunately, not the case. You need to be sexy at all ages.

In the real world, appearances count and continue to count whatever your age, status, health or wealth. And it's much more difficult engaging with people and helping them if they find you physically repulsive.

Malcolm Gladwell's *Blink* tells a series of anecdotes about how we all use what he calls our 'adaptive unconscious' – that part of our brain which leaps to rapid conclusions. In the blink of an eye, we meet a new person and we come to an assessment. Two seconds may be all it takes to decide whether this new person is someone you can like or not. Since humans seem programmed to make snap decisions such as this, isn't it important to appear the best you can be all of the time?

Of course, teenagers and young adults know all about seduction and creating sex appeal. The mating game ensures that they are preoccupied with clothes, make-up, mouthwash and underarm hygiene. But body culture goes well beyond finding a partner in the mindset of the Young Brain.

'Get your mind thinking young and your body will respond ... reject the thinking that it's normal for your joints to start aching, for your belly to hang like a sack of spuds, for the ageing process to overwhelm you. We don't have to do middle age. Many people try to destroy themselves – smoking, alcohol abuse, drugs, unhealthy food, no exercise, stress, suntanning skin damage, negative and anxious mindsets. With a proper lifestyle you can make it healthily to a hundred and enjoy every bit of it.'

Bill Cullen

The result of all of this? Being healthy, fit, strong and supple. Having energy to burn. Experiencing a warm glow inside. Sensing that you are attractive to yourself and others. Feeling a sexual charge. And, most importantly, to feel pride in how you look. You may not be naturally handsome or pretty, but the inner glow will give you a powerful attractiveness.

Just how 'enlightened' is this? Face it: people like, love or respect those whom they find attractive. It is rarish to find a world leader who is not slim and suntanned. Who can argue that Ronald Regan's actorly good looks did not count in his favour? Did Bill Clinton have sex appeal? Would Nelson Mandela have had the same appeal if he had been 50 pounds overweight?

So, once again, the rule is that if you want to do good, first do good to yourself. Self-loathing is not a recipe for being able to help others. Feel good, look good, do good.

Sometimes selfishness spills over into narcissism. This can take many forms but obvious ones include lip enhancements, nose jobs, piercing, scarification and tummy tucks. It is true that some young people get sucked into a fantasy world of self-repair and regeneration. The biology that they were given is reworked by the scalpel of a clever surgeon. Is this wise?

The evidence is that it is a very slippery slope and once you start manipulating your appearance in this way it is hard not to 'just take that up/off'. Then it's something else and yet another nip and tuck. As we said in Chapter 1, this is a superficial approach to youthfulness and nothing more.

The key here, for Young Brains, seems to be authenticity. To be proud of your body, it's got to be yours – and a product of your hard work. Short cuts and superficiality will not deliver the boost to your deep-down self-respect that you – and others – need. Body culture is about being able to be proud of yourself – in preparation for helping others.

Living the Wisdom

To a greater or lesser extent, we all need to de-slob. Try not to say 'Exercise, diet, meditation – I don't do those.' Instead, have a go. Give some things a try and see what sticks. You may find that yoga, or meditation, or cutting down on alcohol has a surprising and significantly positive impact on your sense of well-being.

Stand up for yourself

Young Brains know that, in today's mobile society, friends simply come and go. They also know that strong competition can make the world seem a very aggressive place. This being the case, 'you are your own best friend'.

The concept of enlightened selfishness means something subtly different here. It's about being self-centred enough in order to stick up for yourself, to be kind to yourself, to be caring and nurturing of your soul. It comes from the realisation that, in a bottom-up ultra-competitive society, if you don't look after yourself, no one else is going to. Sad? Yes. An indictment on society? Probably.

You may have witnessed two people arguing loudly and irreverently in public. In polite society, one should not do this. Respect for others and simple good manners mean that backchatting is not permitted.

However, replay the scene from the point of view of self-respect. If another person is being cruel, unfair or vindictive, don't you, as an individual, have the right to stand up for yourself? It's unfortunate if the dispute takes place in full public view, but sometimes you cannot pick the time and place. The blow-up happens and you have to deal with it then and there. Backing off from the argument and saying 'We'll talk later in private' might be taken to indicate that you are not sure of yourself. Better to defend the accusations when they are made.

From a Young Brain's perspective this is all about being sure of what you stand for. It is, once more, about authenticity.

'Authenticity is the key value in the life of young people. This implies more than simply doing your own thing. It means you are real, do not play games or act out a role. You show you are 'real' by adopting clear standpoints. It is always better to have an un-nuanced standpoint than to have no standpoint at all. And artificial is completely unacceptable.'

Adjiedj Bakas, Megatrends Europe

In other words, maybe you'll come across as 'rude' to someone who is easily offended, but it is better to be open and honest and thus to defend your own views than to hold your tongue and slink away. This is lose/lose. You lose self-respect and the adversary loses the opportunity to have his opinions put to the test.

'Delays in explanations give grievances a weight that they would lack if the matter had been addressed as soon as it had arisen. To display anger shortly after an offence occurs is the most generous thing one may do.'

Alain de Botton, *Essays in Love*

Look, it's not that politeness and decorum don't have their place. They do. But if you give them prominence in all situations, you risk being ignored, or even trampled underfoot on occasion.

Like it or not, everyone has to be prepared to stick up for their own interests today, even if this provokes deep-set fears.

'Whenever we take a chance and enter unfamiliar territory or put ourselves into the world in a new way, we experience fear. Very often this fear keeps us from moving ahead with our lives. The trick is to feel the fear and do it anyway.'

Susan Jeffers

Selfishly standing up for yourself and your interests can mean many things. It means knowing your rights – and responsibilities. Having standards, i.e. drawing the line and letting people know when they've overstepped that line. It's about being assertive – knowing what you want and asking for it unambiguously. It can be about complaining, arguing and exiting, as we saw earlier.

It's also about respecting your uniqueness and bringing that to full fruition. It's about treats and rewards for things well done and not being too hard on yourself for things that went wrong. Pampering comes into this too. Why not? You deserve it. You also deserve to be contented and happy. It's not unreasonable to aim to have happiness in your life.

The Young Brain wisdom is to recognise that if you deny yourself, and if you run away from who you really are and what you really need, then you will be less than effective in all your other dealings. To help and care for others, you must start with yourself. You must engage in inner development, body culture and standing up for yourself. Be everything you can be ... and then give some back.

Living the Wisdom

Next time someone tries to trample on you, really irritate them by smiling back. You take away their power, and keep it for yourself. Failing that, go on the offensive. You owe it to yourself to muster your arguments and defend yourself. Do this just once and analyse the results. If positive, go on to another situation where you feel put upon and confront that too. If your attempts to be combative backfire, simply regroup, recalibrate and try again.

Find your emotional nexus

The Old Brain is what social scientists call 'referential', meaning that the Old Brain judges itself in relation to others. In this evaluation, the Old Brain either has higher or lower or similar status versus a given other.

The Young Brain makes fewer such comparisons. It tends to be what psychologists call 'intrinsically' motivated. What matters is not what *others* think, it's your own internal benchmarks and standards, e.g. how comfortable you are with yourself, and how fulfilled you are.

This, then, is part of enlightened selfishness. For the Young Brain, enlightened selfishness is wider than just finding yourself if you've lost your way or lost your sense of self. It's also about developing scores based on internal metrics. Learning, experiencing new feelings, listening to one's emotions – they are all important to developing your YQ, and they are all intrinsic orientations.

The following statistics illustrate how much more young people are intrinsically oriented compared with older cohorts. They actively search out new emotions and are driven by them.

I would like to experience new feelings each day

	15–17	18–24	25–34	35–44	45–54	55–64	65+
% Agree	72	73	64	59	59	54	36

Source: Sociovision 3SC UK, 2005

Developing one's intrinsic orientation is central to Young Brain thinking. If you have watched reality TV programmes, you may have noticed that, when people get voted off, they often say good luck to the remaining participants and follow it up with the advice 'Be true to yourself.' This may not sound revolutionary but it means, for example, that the Young Brain is more emotional, intuitive and inner-directed. The Young Brain shouts, cries and wears its feelings on its sleeve.

This goes against the grain of the Old Brain and, as a result, watching reality TV can be quite alarming to the Old Brain. Given that an Old Brain values what others think and tries to be constant and unemotional whatever the circumstances, it finds this raw emotion very disturbing – particularly when it is grown men doing the crying.

We call this aspect of the Young Brain its 'emotional nexus'. The nexus, or link between cause and effect, means internal feelings channel directly through to external expressions of emotions. As a result, Young Brains tend to be more frank in exchanges with other people – rather like the extremely direct way people talk to each other in soap operas.

Why is the emotional nexus part of the Wisdom of Youth? Simply, because it liberates people to be real human beings.

'We all have feelings, so why hide them?' says the Young Brain. Ignore what others think, forget status and forget the shell that we build around our emotions as we get older. Emotions are good; they help us feel alive, they tap into our intuitions and innate sensing mechanisms. They give Young Brains an intrinsic orientation.

Living the Wisdom

Next time you see someone crying in public (for example, a sportsperson who just failed) refuse to see him or her as a double looser. Give others the benefit of the doubt and look upon their reactions as an honest expression of apology. Be more forgiving of others' emotions and soon you'll be more open emotionally yourself.

3 Helping others

Helping others challenges

1 When did you last put your needs ahead of someone crying for all of your attention – and feel you were doing the right thing?

2 Are you currently undertaking an activity where you can really claim to be making a difference in the life of someone less fortunate than yourself?

If you gave answers that were not entirely convincing, then read on and find out how to adopt a 'helping others' mindset.

Be selfish first

Enlightened selfishness is crucial for everyone who wants to recapture their youth. However, it has particular relevance for a specific group of people – those spending a significant part of their day looking after the welfare of others.

Giving service to others – whether it's parenting, teaching, caring, or one of the myriad forms of helping and supporting – is both meaningful and worthwhile. At the same time it is essentially unselfish, other-oriented and, taken to the extreme, can leave the helper feeling lonely and uncared for.

So enlightened selfishness recognises that giving humanely while losing your own humanity is the wrong strategy. It is important to put aside some time and invest some effort in considering yourself, and your own emotional needs as an individual. Only then can you give your best to others.

For people given to being utterly selfless, this is a challenging wisdom. But, although it can at first be somewhat jarring, realise that it's important for three reasons.

Firstly, it reduces the temptation to use service to others as an excuse for not paying attention to your own mental and emotional freshness and development. It is all too easy to let physical appearance slip, and almost relish being a bit frumpy and uncool.

Secondly, investing time and effort in yourself allows you both to keep growing as a human being and to confirm your individuality and your attractiveness.

Thirdly, the confidence you gain through growing and developing enables you to engage more effectively with those around you. You have more energy, more insight and more courage.

The Wisdom of Youth knows that the best way to love others is to love oneself. It's like the airlines' injunctions to passengers in case of a sudden loss of air pressure to put on their own oxygen mask before they help their children. You can help others more effectively if you are functioning on all emotional cylinders yourself.

Or look at it this way. If you invest heavily in your vegetable patch and have a bumper harvest, chances are everyone benefits. Neighbours, friends and family – everyone gets a few potatoes, radishes and tomatoes. Likewise, Young Brains can give more, once they have harvested the fruits of their own self-development.

This is not about self-indulgence and vanity. It is about autonomy and fulfilment. Young people do it naturally. But, as we get older, we sometimes need to discipline ourselves to be selfish in this enlightened way, in order for us to fulfil our potential as human beings.

In essence, this means refreshing your *view* of your self. Old Brains tend to take themselves for granted. Once you begin to fully appreciate the value you add to life around you, and the richness of talents, attitudes and skills you bring to the party, you will find you will be able to refresh and re-energise those capabilities, i.e. you will adopt Young Brain thinking.

Living the Wisdom

Hard-wire some 'ME' time into your day. Get a dog and take it for walks; close the door and meditate for 15 minutes; turn off the car CD when you drive. Use this bubble of time to think about yourself, what your body and brain are saying and your needs. Once you've properly listened to yourself, next develop and implement some actions to support your own 'child within'.

Social philanthropy

Our theme incorporates 'enlightenment' for a very good reason. *Serviam*, Latin for 'I will serve', is a moto needed as never before.

In developed societies up to 70 per cent of women work and so necessarily have to reduce caring concerns. Meanwhile, governments around the world are tightening social security budgets. So what happens to children, to the poor, the needy, the weak and the infirm in this brave new world? The less advantaged in our society need individuals to be enlightened to take up the slack.

The need for charitable help is huge, and the demand for carers is growing rapidly. Western societies are ageing, and putting elderly people into care homes is becoming less affordable for both individuals and governments. The requirement for long-term care in the domestic home is therefore rising at an alarming rate. Some projections for the UK estimate that well over half the households in the country will have one of the members in them acting as a carer by 2020.

Volunteering is a Young Brained activity and seems to be getting more and more popular among the young (although plenty of older people get involved, because, as we shall see in the last chapter, this also touches on the wisdom of experience). Young Brains want to make an impression on the world in which they live. *Wanting to make a difference is about desiring to be someone, to be effective as a human being, to make life a little better for others.* Researchers in America conclude that college student volunteering increased by approximately 20 per cent between 2002 and 2005.

And, generally speaking, you wouldn't do it unless you enjoyed it and got satisfaction from it.

Beyond volunteering and getting involved in charity events and activities, Young Brains also tend to be in the front line on other social issues. They organise grassroots protest movements, and they get involved with non-government organisations (NGOs) of all kinds. Young Brains are also in the vanguard of bringing environmental issues to the fore – something Old Brains are taking time coming to terms with.

If you want something done, ask a busy person. Better still, ask a Young Brain.

Older brains tend to have given up on the desire to be different, to do things differently and make a difference. And when they do seek change it is more likely to be focused on personal social climbing. As we said, Old Brains are referential, and tend to get hooked on social status. When your thinking is driven by where you fit in the economic system, philanthropy tends to focus on giving money (recognised by a plaque or your name on a hospital ward) rather than time (little recognition because you're just one of many volunteers and cameras can't be present all the time). Volunteering earns no money and the satisfactions are intrinsic, earning little public recognition.

'The character of a man can be judged by his dealing with people who cannot possibly do him any favours.'

Johann von Goethe, 1749–1832

Old Brains no longer believe that what they do will have the slightest effect on the world around them and focus more on their own social standing. Young Brains, by contrast, fight every step of the way for their right to be heard, to challenge the status quo and change the world.

There is also a bonus in store for altruistic Young Brains. Volunteering to help others is proven in studies to keep you young – even in extreme old age.

'Research amongst over 600 Community Service Volunteers (the UK's largest volunteering and training organisation) showed that there are direct physical and mental health benefits in volunteering. Not only is volunteers' mental health better, they take less sick days, and even enjoy noticeable weight loss.'

Tim Drake, *I Want to Make a Difference*

This is another of those virtuous circles. Young Brains want to make a difference and, by helping others, they stay Young Brains. A real win:win.

Living the Wisdom

Think through what social or environmental concerns you are passionate about and volunteer for unpaid work. It just comes down to making contact and getting involved. Nothing more, nothing less. The principle is well captured by Oxfam's slogan on the volunteering page of its website: 'Yourself: Please give generously.'

SUMMARY OF GOALS

Enlightened selfishness is crucial to embracing the Young Brain mindset. It regenerates your pride in yourself and your enthusiasm for life. It also gives you the clear conscience and the physical breathing room to make progress on this and other Wisdoms.

The goals for this Wisdom are:

- Acknowledge you have power and be prepared to use it.
- Work on improving your self-esteem; get a bird's-eye view of the strengths you bring to the party.
- Help others by first helping yourself and then giving something back through volunteering or caring activities.

Feeling more positive about yourself already? Excellent. You'll have to work constantly at this one, as we all find that the demons of self-doubt are always trying to step back in. This chapter may need revisiting more than most.

But we can't stop now – it's on to the next Wisdom: Fresh Blood.

05

Fresh Blood

Luckily the young Russian twins had each other to talk to. They had arrived at their new school in Milan halfway through the first term. Their teacher was concerned for them. Not only had they been uprooted and brought to a new country, they could speak no Italian, and their classmates had already formed their own groupings and friendships.

Inga and Klara, after early uncertainty, laughed and got on with it. They joined in, talking to the other children in Russian, until they had enough Italian words to make themselves understood. A few months later they each had their own friends, and their teacher was delighted with their progress. In particular, she was thrilled by their ability to bond with their classmates, despite their language difficulties.

The Russian twins exhibited Young Brain behaviour at its most natural and inclusive. By being open and engaging they had turned around a potentially hostile and alienating situation – and come away with life-enhancing personal growth.

It is a sad irony that many Old Brains – even speaking in their mother tongue – remain distant and cold when they find themselves in a new social setting. They feel threatened by outside groups or strangers. Only within their own social circle do they feel comfortable. They need to learn another wisdom from youth. They need a Fresh Blood mindset.

Defining 'Fresh Blood'

This chapter is about bringing new people – fresh blood – into your social circle. Indeed, it's about dissolving the idea of a social circle, and creating an openness to other people that is without boundaries. It means making friends frequently and easily. It means being more trusting and less cynical concerning strangers. It also means being less bashful and more extroverted.

Being open to people offers the possibilities of new friendships that may not just reinvigorate you personally but also your old friendships. Adding someone new and interesting to the gene pool of your social friendships and acquaintances can transform everyday life. Relationships that were subsiding gently into atrophy can come alive. Just bringing in fresh blood, with fresh stories and ideas, can make social intercourse altogether more enlivened and interesting.

'If a man does not make new acquaintance as he advances through life, he will soon find himself alone. A man, Sir, should keep his friendship in constant repair.'
Dr Samuel Johnson (1709–1794)

Don't worry, we won't be asking you to give up your friends. Just to get to a stage where you genuinely enjoy meeting and engaging with strangers. It's all part of how Young Brains have more fun and stimulating experiences compared with Old Brains.

Fresh blood is about sociability but (like enlightened selfishness) it's also about personal attractiveness and maybe even sex appeal. You see, how we relate to others comes down to how interested you are in other people, and also how interesting and appealing you are, in turn, to them. Whatever insecurities you may have felt in the past on this front, if you engage wholeheartedly with each 'Living the Wisdom' these doubts will soon fall away; your confidence and self-esteem will grow, and the attractive and interesting person inside you will blossom for all to see.

Accepting others

It is striking just how much our openness to others reduces with age. The following table from a British social survey reveals a very high correlation between our openness to others and our chronological age.

I am part of several networks of people

	15–17	18–24	25–34	35–44	45–54	55–64	65+
% Agree	51	48	42	42	35	45	32

Source: Sociovision 3SC UK, 2005

As we get older, we tend to turn away from others and multiple networks. The fall-off has started even by the time we reach 18, and the declines are most steep after the short burst of sociability that often follows retirement.

Young people are the most sociable – as any parent who has to pay their kids' monthly mobile phone bills will testify. This comes naturally to them, just as it did to the Russian twins. However, Young Brains continue to be gregarious – be they 30 or 60 years old. You probably know people like this. You cannot sit with them for more than half an hour without their phone ringing several times. People are always popping in for a chat. Like flowers attract bees, they are always humming. And the pay-off of all this socialising is massive.

Benefits of Fresh Blood

Just look at some of the benefits:

● Helping you be connected and informed.

- Keeping you interested and interesting – even sexy.

- Bringing in fresh ideas and up-to-date information.

- Giving you new outlooks on life; shaking things up.

- Allowing you learn more about yourself – and your partner.

- Stimulating comfortable old friendships and keeping everyone on their toes.

- Reducing dependency on your existing circle of close friends or family.

- Helping you to feel less isolated and alone in the twilight years, as old friends shuffle off this mortal coil.

- Replacing the loss of social network when your kids leave home, and you lose contact with their friends and the kids-oriented social functions.

- Liberating you to make substantive changes in your life (if you make friends naturally, a physical relocation, for example, will feel less threatening to your equilibrium).

Don't become a recluse

We all know about celebrity recluses such as Howard Hughes or Greta Garbo who famously said 'I want to be let alone.' Unfortunately, the world is populated by millions living lonely lives of quiet desperation. In a world of 6.7 billion people, feeling unloved, isolated and alone is one of life's worse tortures.

How does this happen? How is it possible to go from being surrounded by schoolmates, then work colleagues, to feelings that only a few would care if you went absent without leave?

The answer, once again, comes down to the drift towards Old Brainhood. Rather than keep our social lives interesting and vibrant, we relax and say, 'That's enough, from now on I'll just preserve what I have. I've got enough friends, so why look for others?'

We also start to lose our ability to take risks – and for many nothing feels quite a risky as engaging with strangers.

Finally, Old Brains can start to be stubborn. They tend towards a take-me-as-you-find-me attitude to social relationships which, roughly translated, means, 'I'm not interested in you enough to make an effort to talk with you.' No wonder they can struggle to add to their friendship network.

Avoiding the danger of becoming a recluse is what this wisdom is all about. Just as in the previous two chapters, it will involve challenges to your values and stepping outside of your comfort zones. And, just as in Chapters 3 and 4, it's about adopting new mindsets.

Adopt three Fresh Blood mindsets as your own

When it comes to forming new relationships, Young Brains tend to think in ways that are different from Middle-aged and Old Brains. Young Brains welcome Fresh Blood into their lives by:

1 connecting with others
2 crowd belonging
3 building trust.

Let's look at each of them in turn.

1 Connecting with others

Connecting challenges

1 How many new people have you met and kept in contact with over the last 3 months?

2 How many friends do you have who are from totally different social or racial backgrounds from yourself?

3 Do you count people who are substantially younger than you as friends?

How did you do? If your answers left you feeling you may have some work to do in this area, that's fine. The following Young Brain attitudes should set you on the road to a more rewarding and enjoyable social scene.

Charisma not class

We are moving slowly towards an entirely new era in the way we structure society. Time was when many relationships were determined by social class. In former times, if you were born into the same social class, racial group or caste as me, then I'd talk to you as an equal. If not, then we were unlikely to be friends. The powerful forces keeping these boundaries in place are captured in books such as Forster's *A Room with a View*. And again in films such as Cameron's *Titanic*, where the ocean liner is not the only thing to hit a hard place. Rose's need for human warmth equally hits the iceberg called social convention.

Today, in many societies around the world, this particular page is turning. Class isn't what it used to be. Deference – forelock-tugging to authority – is now mostly reserved for celebrities and, sometimes, royalty. Those in upper classes no longer automatically command respect. They have to earn it. In today's society we become respected for who we are because of what we do, not by virtue of what class we were born into. This changes everything.

For Young Brains, rather than a breakdown in social order, this levelling – sometimes called the democratisation of society – is a very positive thing. It means, for example, that anyone could potentially become their friend. What matters is whether you do the same things, go to the same places and who cares about the rest? Born into another class? Irrelevant. Have a different colour skin? So what?

The progressive loss of social convention and social etiquette has other important consequences. Fewer arranged marriages, for example, and fewer 'coming out' balls. All of a sudden, it's charisma that counts. Who you are as a person, and what you do with your life become the keys to social success; not social standing. Once again, it's game on for everyone.

Old Brains find this new, flatter world hard to accept – or even see. They say pompous things such as 'I'm head of the committee, you know' and believe that they've said enough to win them friends and influence. As bosses, they believe that they will find friends because those around will be in awe of their power. In the economic hierarchy, they hold on to the traditional notion that money can buy anything – including friendship.

The truth is that, nowadays, personality and not rank, or where you live, is what is important if you want a vibrant social network. Finding fresh blood is more about being *interesting* and less about being important.

Living the Wisdom

From now on, do your best to befriend interesting people (rather than 'powerful' people). If someone makes you laugh, stimulates your creative juices or gets you going intellectually, go out of your way to be friendly and spend more time with them.

Be informal and approachable

Here are some questions for you. Are you able to open up to a shop assistant spontaneously and chummily when asking for advice in a store? When was the last time you were able to quite naturally start talking to the lady in the window seat on a plane? And, while you are waiting in a queue, do you cross your arms and frown in a 'don't-you-dare-even-try-to-talk-to-me' pose?

It is quite possible that you still blush when strangers talk to you. Moreover, you might confess that introducing yourself to others still brings you out in a metaphorical – even a physical – sweat. In both cases, you'll want to become more informal and approachable.

If you do feel uncomfortable with others, this is probably one of the bigger tasks of this book. We know that. Yes, you want to become youthful but, you say, can't that just sidestep having to interact with strangers? Is this you? If it is, the comforting message is that, no, you don't have to do everything recommended by this book. We all have Achilles heels and pushing on with other wisdoms which don't bring you out in cold sweats is the right approach.

However, that's no excuse for many others who just let themselves off the hook too easily. A little more effort and confidence and they would be there. Young Brains use informality and approachability to help them cross the invisible line between a cold distancing with a stranger and a warm welcoming approach. The kind of contact that implicitly says: 'I don't know you, but it is possible we could become friends.'

Living the Wisdom

We know it's tough, but next time you are facing a stranger in a railway carriage or similar situation, gather up your willpower and open up a conversation, stay informal and most of all be approachable. Success is when the other person responds warmly to you (probably sometime after the initial exchange). Congratulate your younger self by treating your Young Brain to a sticky cake and coffee when you arrive at your station!

Make the most of mobility

Chances are that your grandfather and grandmother came from the same town or village. Your parents may have travelled further afield but, probably, they still married someone from the same region, race and religion.

But, today, provoked by a couple of decades of high mobility, we find marriages and civil partnerships that blend races, blur national cultures and mix religions. As we zip from pillar to post for our jobs and our social lives, this super-mobility pushes Young Brains to be open to others – other races, other creeds and other cultures.

Why? Because by meeting strangers every day of every week of every month, the scales of prejudice and ignorance begin to fall from people's eyes. The foreign becomes accepted, and the alien becomes normal. Where initially you saw only the colour of the skin, or someone's faith, as you get to know them, they become just Jo, or Mahalia, Shaku or Abe. They are human beings you know and like, not racial or religious stereotypes.

Constantly encountering people from different ethnic or social backgrounds becomes stimulating. It enriches social intercourse. For Young Brains living in cities where the ethnic and social mixes are more varied and colourful, going back to single-origin friendships would be both monochrome and dull.

One simple measure of physical mobility is the amount of international travel. Take Britain: in 2006 just under 33 million people arrived on its shores. That's a lot of fresh blood. Meanwhile, UK residents made 66 million visits abroad. That's a lot of opportunities to make new friends.

Given this global melting pot, older brains, which refuse to embrace others, cut themselves off from a potpourri of rich experience. More importantly, perhaps, they are refusing to recognise the multicultural world as it is today. Being open to others – whatever their origin – is a fundamental necessity if we are to feel at ease in our contemporary world.

No-one can deny the huge social shifts created by increasing physical mobility. Young Brains recognise this, celebrate it and join in. Their connectivity flourishes as a consequence.

Living the Wisdom

Work on making friends from diverse cultural backgrounds. Ensure that your friends are not just local and that you are in regular contact with people living in other countries. Holidays are great opportunities for this – but only if the obligatory exchange of addresses at the end of the vacation leads to being in rapid contact once back home! With texts, messaging, Facebook and emails, none of us has any more excuses not to do so.

Deploy new networking possibilities

We live in a networked society where we are increasingly connected, principally via new technologies such as the mobile phone and Internet.

The number of people connected to the Internet via a computer or a mobile device grows by the minute. And the explosion of mobile phones means that some countries have more mobile users than fixed line users. BlackBerries, and variations thereof, are omnipresent on trains and planes around the world. It often seems that at least a third of all people waiting for their bags at airports are chatting on the phone, receiving emails, surfing the web or texting home. Evolving wireless technologies means laptops will soon be online 24/7. Or whatever replaces laptops.

In such a connected information-rich world, Young Brains know that they have to be 'always on' (we come back to this in the next chapter). They are ready to strike up a conversation with anybody at any time. This has stimulated – and confirmed – the desire to go *towards* others rather than retreat into the comfort zone of old friends and acquaintances.

In a recent US survey, women spent 453 minutes a month chatting on their mobile phones whilst men … well, men spent longer – 458 minutes a month gabbing on their mobiles. Women, though, spend more time on fixed phones at home – another 455 minutes a month. That represents, over 15 hours of chat per month – or a full 3% of their waking lives talking to others on the phone.

AT&T, www.att.com

Any reader with an adolescent (or even pre-adolescent) son or daughter will probably see this as small in comparison to what they witness on a daily basis. No wonder we say that technology is facilitating our openness to others.

For the Young Brain, these technical advances are not merely mechanisms which accelerate and facilitate communication between people. They have led to both tighter bonds and broader networks. This is the new culture of connectivity.

Ask a Young Brain what it is doing when it telephones, for example, and you might be surprised by the answer. Often, it's not about transmitting information at all – rather, it's about *conveying one's emotions in real time*. For example, a Young Brain might say 'I'm on the bus,' but what is *really* being communicated is 'I'm really excited about our night on the town.'

Meanwhile, anyone who's witnessed young people doing a 'thumb dance' on the keypad of their mobile phones or BlackBerry's as they send texts and emails back and forth will know the buzz that comes from this new kind of real-time dialoguing.

Communicating emotions like this in a stream of consciousness creates much tighter bonds with close friends than the Old Brain could ever imagine. Being 'always on' means being 'always there' – and what more could you want from your best friends than that?

This is not to say that writing letters, for example, is not an elegant and intimate way of relating to friends. But when you pour your heart out in a letter, your friends' empathetic best wishes and advice will take several days to find their way back to you. By which time, you may be on another emotional plane altogether.

Conversely, almost guaranteed instant access to your best mate, via his or her mobile, when you feel like crying your eyes out ensures that you get the fillip at the moment it's most needed. From this, deeper friendships are born.

As we said, the culture of connectivity is about deeper relationships – and also broader relationships. New multiple networks of belonging mean that Young Brains ramp up more weakly bonded relationships than the Old Brain could ever contemplate.

An Old Brain often will have a few friends and a few dozen acquaintances. The Young Brain, in this new technologically enabled world, has hundreds – or even thousands – of contacts.

As anyone with a MySpace page, or an entry on FaceBook, will know, contacts are very easy to come by.

Malcolm Gladwell says some people shy away from the casual cultivation of acquaintances saying: 'we have our circle of friends, to whom we are devoted. Acquaintances we keep at arm's length ... we don't want to feel obliged to have dinner with them ... or visit them when they are sick. The purpose of making an acquaintance, for most of us, is to evaluate whether we want to turn that person into a friend.' The people described here have Old Brain reasoning.

Gladwell encounters other people who have, he reckons, mastered the 'weak tie' – i.e. the ability to make a friendly yet casual social connection. He has his own term for these people – he calls them 'connectors'. Connectors display the Wisdom of Youth for they: 'manage to occupy many different worlds and subcultures and niches ... a function of something intrinsic to their ... curiosity, self-confidence, sociability and energy'.

Malcolm Gladwell, *The Tipping Point*

Rather than dismissing the superficiality of chat rooms and Internet friendships, we must think through the advantages. The capacity to accept and develop a multitude of acquaintances spills out into the real world. What we are saying is that there are now different ways to attract fresh blood which set a new pace, and that these need to be considered – and acted upon – by people who want to prevent their brains from ageing.

Connecting to others opens a wealth of opportunities for the Young Brain. It keeps life fresh and friendly.

If you are not already doing so, shouldn't you connect today?

2 Crowd belonging

Crowd belonging challenges

1 How often did you go out with a whole group of friends over the last three months?

2 How many different social networks (associations, clubs, rather distinct groups of friends, etc.) do you belong to?

Surprised by your answers? Don't worry. You have chosen to read this book because you want to do things differently in your life. You want to rejuvenate. Feeling confident in a crowd is part of the solution.

Seek out collective emotions

Young Brains are at ease with crowds. They enjoy both the vibrant diversity found in a large public gathering and the outpouring of collective emotions. We call this a desire for crowd belonging.

Of course, not everyone enjoys crowds – and you may be one of these. Crowds can be noisy and dirty; they attract 'all sorts'.

They can be promiscuous or dangerous. You can get physically jostled and barged about and feel claustrophobic. Why would anyone go out of their way to be pressed up against the masses?

However, if you do find yourself shying away from crowds, think again. People who say: 'I don't go here/I try not to go there, because there are just too many people' have an older brain mentality. And this slide into older thinking starts in our twenties. Young Brains have a good time in crowds, as the following data show.

I like to have a good time in a crowd

	15–17	18–24	25–34	35–44	45–54	55–64	65+
% Agree	75	74	65	58	51	47	29

Source: Sociovision 3SC UK, 2005

The consequences of these attitudes is witnessed by the explosion of music festivals of all kinds over the last ten years. In Britain, the most famous music festivals have traditionally included Glastonbury, Reading and the Isle of Wight. More recently, so many others have popped up that, increasingly, today's talk is of saturation.

But the drive to enjoy yourself among lots of other people is not limited to music, of course. We can add major sporting events, theme parks, exhibitions and demonstrations to the list. Think back to recent mass events – the 9/11 five-year commemorations, Live 8, the ten-year memorial concert for Diana, Princess of Wales, the concert for Mandela at 90, and the story is clear. Crowds have a strong appeal. Why?

Participating in mass gatherings signals many things. It says you are happy with humanity and that you respect your fellow citizens. It shows you trust others (we'll come back to this shortly) and believe that they will trust you. Most importantly, it also highlights your yearning for collective emotions.

The Young Brain knows that mass gatherings are rare moments, which, in the right circumstances, can truly connect them with their emotions. And not just 'ordinary' emotions but 'collective' emotions that they cannot experience in any other way.

In 2002 Queen Elizabeth II celebrated her Golden Jubilee. There was a party at the Palace for 12,000 invitees, which included a spectacular music concert and, for the public, a celebration was planned for The Mall. Organisers forecast several hundreds of thousands would attend, but were overwhelmed to see an estimated 1 million turn up to dance the afternoon and evening away. Were these all fervent monarchists? Clearly not. Many were simply Young Brains seeking a party and an emotional high by 'feeling part of it'.

Have you ever experienced this? To say collective emotions are strong feelings would be to underestimate them. They usually manifest themselves as sensations of bonding, peace and being at one with mankind. The emotional outpouring can be spiritual in nature or sometimes be highly sexually charged.

A recent survey of attitudes of people shopping in London's West End showed a striking difference between age groups. For older shoppers, Oxford Street and other central shopping thoroughfares were to be avoided at all costs. Why? The transport was congested, the pavements were cluttered, and the shops were crowded. Ghastly.

Young shoppers, conversely, welcomed all these things. What was a living hell for the silver shoppers was a living heaven for the youth. They delighted in the vibrancy, energy and rich diversity of London's Carnaby Street and Covent Garden. And, rather than being put off by the crowds, they were a validation and a legitimisation of their choice of place to shop. It was an 'in' place because others like them had also chosen it. They could tap into positive collective emotions.

Living the Wisdom

Take time out to ask some teenagers or young adults just what they get from being in a crowd and why it is important for them to go to mass gatherings. Be prepared to be open-minded. Ask yourself the question: 'Am I missing out on something rather exhilarating and liberating?'

Find friends in crowds

Social research has shown that the way we go about choosing our friends has changed. Today, it is less about principle and much more about practice. In other words, we are most likely to choose friends because they do the same things as I do and go to the same places that I go to rather than because they share the same attitudes or values.

Think about this a minute. It means you find friends through your activities, your work, your play, your associative life, rather than through, for example, your class or your attitudes. Here we echo a theme we picked up earlier in the chapter.

Of course, talk to older brains and they will tell you that, to get on with others, you need to share ideals; it is important to see eye to eye on important ideological issues such as politics, religion and morality. So, if you found yourself slightly incredulous about the research results above, it is, unfortunately, your Old Brain whispering in your ear.

The fact is that Young Brains need less and less to feel they have to agree with the values of their friends. Indeed, a healthy disagreement once in a while about trade unions, gay rights or ecological concerns is perhaps exactly what is needed to keep a friendship bubbling.

The Wisdom of Youth says, therefore, forget trying to agree with your friends on values and beliefs. It is OK to have contrary points of view and still be friends. This has enormous implications for friendship. For example, it opens up your friendship circle to include millions of individuals you fundamentally disagree with!

Of course, we are not saying that values no longer count – only that they matter less when it comes to filtering possible friends. Opposites really do attract.

Looking at the flip side, you will find more friends the more things you do. Sounds obvious, doesn't it? Get out and about, join more networks and you are sure to meet fresh blood. And since going to the same places is key, one of the potentially most fertile places to make new acquaintances is in a crowd. Indeed, this is another reason why crowd belonging is such a strong emotion. You are sharing a place, a time and an event with others. And you could easily make friends as a consequence.

Incidentally, don't think that advertisers have ignored such analysis. Look at how many outdoor events are sponsored by big brands today. Whether rock festivals, opera by the lake, marathons or charity fun runs, marketers know that collective emotions and new friendship ties make a potent mixture. 'Get them when they have opened their minds to outside influences and when they are emotionally charged.' If crowds are open to making friends, then let my brand be a friend which also shows up.

The sponsorship of stadia is further evidence of this – look at the 'O2' Millennium Dome, or Arsenal's Emirates football ground and the Washington Redskins' FedexField stadium.

And, of course, charity events are also great places to make new friends. Indeed, social research into volunteering for charity fundraising reveals that one important reason for getting involved is to generate a social life. It gets you out of the house and into the arms of a welcoming and passionate group of activists.

Meanwhile, the charity events that are organised by the volunteers can themselves be a tremendous source of collective emotions. For example, Cancer Research UK's Race for Life has runners with cards pinned to their chests commemorating the special person they lost to cancer. It doesn't get more poignant than that.

In addition, mass charity events such as Red Nose Day show that fundraising can also be fun-raising.

In short, Young Brains revel in the big crowd frisson, interaction, communal emotion, and friendships that form, and the fact that diverse peoples come together in harmony. Follow their lead and let crowd belonging create new meaning in your life.

Living the Wisdom

Start getting out into the crowds, and enjoying the buzz of a big event. Be alert, find out what's going on and, for once, forget about penny-pinching. Events can be expensive but this is an investment in your future – and your youthfulness.

Enjoy it, and take the opportunity to be open to new people and, potentially, new friends.

If there are no big events coming up, create your own crowd. Throw a party or invite a whole group of people to the pub next Friday evening.

3 Building trust

Trust challenges

1 Are you able to be entirely yourself when you are with your friends and feel you can let down your guard?

2 If a motorcyclist was knocked off his bike outside your home, would you invite him inside until he had recovered his wits?

Poll after poll demonstrate that we are losing trust in our institutions and in the powers that be. Journalists, politicians, even doctors and scientists suffer from declining levels of public confidence. But, if you were to take from this that cynicism is rife everywhere, you'd be wrong. Young Brains show high levels of trust. Indeed, to introduce fresh blood into your life, you absolutely have to give others, at some stage, the benefit of the doubt. You have to be able to both trust others and to build trust with them.

An inability to trust can make you friendless and sad throughout your whole life.

Open up

Since human relationships are highly uncertain, trust becomes key. For, in friendship, just as in love, there is no formal contract enforceable by law. You cannot force someone to like or love you.

For a relationship to be authentic, therefore, you must give friendship without consideration of what you might get in return.

'Trust must lie at the heart of true communicative friendship in the contemporary world. There are no rules and contracts to bind us to our closest friends: we simply have to trust them. Without trust, friendships will fail.'

Raymond Pahl, *On Friendship*

Trust has many manifestations. One of the most important, in this context, is the confidence to open up to others. Of course, we must go in with our eyes open; we have to recognise that the more we open up, the more others are able to betray us. And yet, trust means having confidence that others will not exploit our nakedness nor our overtures. The only contract between friends is a contract of the heart.

This was recently observed on a London bus. A very attractive young lady started a genuine and friendly conversation with a middle-aged man. Here clearly was a Young Brain in action – spontaneous, authentic and very trusting that her intentions would not be misinterpreted. She got off the bus some stops later with just a friendly 'G'bye'. The point is that she acted in such an open way because her experience over and over again has shown that talking to strangers is a *rewarding* – not a dangerous – thing to do.

Now we are not suggesting that you throw caution to the wind. If you have reason to be suspicious of someone and your antennae are quivering with an instinctive warning of danger, then, of course, step very carefully. But as a general rule be confident that others are nice, generous human beings who, themselves, are looking for a bit of human warmth and friendship. And, if someone opens up to you, respond with enthusiasm, not cynicism.

'Whether we like it or not, we have all been born on this earth as part of one great human family. Rich or poor, educated or uneducated, belonging to one nation or another, to one religion or another, adhering to this ideology or that, ultimately each of us is just a human being like everyone else: we all desire happiness and do not want suffering.'

The Dalai Lama

Trusting others opens up whole new horizons and opportunities. So, let a complete unknown sleep on your sofa for five days? Why not, because they have also signed up to couchsurfing.com? And they'd allow you to do the same on their couch. Swop houses for your three-week summer holiday? Absolutely! There's a whole industry spawned to do just this. Open up your home for a clothes-swapping party. Why not?

Most Old Brains, unfortunately, see things differently. The Old Brains fear that even responding to someone opening a conversation will place some sort of unlooked-for responsibility on their shoulders. They feel that their interlocutor must want something from them. To lead them somewhere they don't want to go. Much safer to say nothing or, if pressurised, to talk about the weather.

For Young Brains, saying nothing is not an option. In fact, they would rather go to the other extreme and let it all hang out. Wearing your emotions on your sleeve and being true to yourself is an integral part of Young Brainhood. This is also a trust factor. By exposing yourself in front of others, Young Brains have confidence that such emotional nakedness will be respected and, possibly, reciprocated.

There's an old expression which says 'People who never get drunk in front of others have something to hide.' While alcohol abuse is not to be condoned, it is one illustration of how Young Brains trusts other Young Brains. Getting legless with your friends demonstrates how comfortable you are with them; almost anything you do and say will not be turned against you in the morning. And you wouldn't dream of mentioning your friend's indiscretions, either – give or take a tad of teasing!

Having said that, Young Brains are not trusting of everyone. For example, Young Brains distrust those who practise emotional control and keeping passions pent up – this strikes them as artificial and shows that the (Older Brained) person is hiding things. This is significant and marks a huge shift in how today's society evaluates others. As we saw earlier, to demonstrate a stiff upper lip was to be trustworthy and dependable in all circumstances. Now, reining in emotions is treated with the utmost suspicion. Being open to others means having no secrets. It means less hypocrisy and more authenticity.

Living the Wisdom

If you have problems opening up, try this. Next time you are away from home, take a trip in a taxi and be more loose-mouthed than you would ever dream of being normally. See where it leads you and monitor how you feel. Maybe feel guilty afterwards – but at least you tried. But maybe, just maybe you'll feel liberated and more willing to engage in intensive, trusting talk with friends closer to home.

Of course, hairdressers and beauticians can often serve the same purpose but frequently the surroundings are less private and the boutique 'too close to home'.

Privacy keeps you a prisoner

The flip side of opening up is keeping private. Keeping your nose out of other people's affairs used to be preached by polite parents. 'Keep yourself to yourself' and 'Mind your own business' were the rules of the road. How life has changed!

Interestingly, female brains are younger than male brains in this respect. Women tend to care more about people and are more interested in them. They remember the names of other people's children, know what age they are and what stage of life they have reached. They talk about people, what they are doing and what issues they are facing, because to them it is important. Women think me-we.

When two male Middle-aged Brains get together, it is not mostly to talk about their personal lives, nor the personal lives of others. The subject is more likely to be which team will win the next match, or what phone they have just purchased. Boys' toys figure large in the conversations of male mates. It comes as a big shock when one of them learns from his own wife that his friend is on the brink of divorce.

This could never happen to a Young Brain – of either sex. 'Indiscretion' (although it's absolutely not seen as that) means having it out, speaking your mind, expecting others to speak theirs. Little is taboo. From the size of your bank account to the size of your … well, you fill in the gap! Young Brains understand that the concept of nosiness is just nonsense.

They also understand that being coy, private and reserved will keep you a prisoner inside your own head. Finding fresh blood is about exchange with others, not keeping to you own company and sacrificing yourself to a stoical life.

Living the Wisdom

Make it your practice always to follow up when a friend drops 'self-revelation' into a conversation. If someone is prepared to be open enough to reveal something heartfelt, your friendship is only worth something if you question him or her about what he or she has just said.

By the way, often and especially where men are concerned, the self-revelation will be hard to detect unless you are really listening to him or her (as you should be). For example, someone (who, in this example, is a person who normally has money to spare) might say, almost in passing, 'Oh, I'd like to join you but I don't think I can afford it.' A concerned friend would pick up on this and ask what had changed and had they recently got into financial difficulties.

Being informed

And here's a big point. We increasingly trust 'people like us' for our information input. Sales staff, scientists, advertisers, politicians, journalists – all fall further down the trust tree than our friends and acquaintances. Why have blogs suddenly become popular? Why do advertisers now invest in viral marketing? Why have message boards, chat rooms and wikinomics all blossomed? It's because, increasingly, we take our information and make our decisions on the basis of input from our network of 'people like me'.

Want to buy an MP3 player? Your brother-in-law is the real expert – not the shop salesman. Want to stop the swelling? Your friend's friend will know the suitable homoeopathic cure better than your doctor. Want to buy a new Toyota? Comments from Toyota owners on car message boards will be more frank than those you'll find on the official Toyota website.

You probably already know the biggest reason people give for switching from one brand to another: low price. But running this a close second is 'advice from my close network'. Being persuaded by advertising or mailings comes well down the list.

Now remember, 'people like me' does not necessarily refer to others who share my attitudes or beliefs. As already said, it's more about people who visit the same places. And by places, we are also talking about virtual locations, i.e. the same websites, chatrooms, noticeboards, etc.

The important thing to note in all of this is that it is the Young Brains who are in the vanguard of the culture of connectivity. Middle-aged and Old Brains are being left behind badly – and missing out on a lot of what society has to offer. For example, Old Brains still go to the authority figures for information well before their family and friends. But accessing knowledge from the upper rungs of the hierarchy can be both frustrating and time consuming. If you have you ever tried to get your laptop computer fixed over the phone using a technical helpline, you know what we are talking about.

Yet knowledge is so decentralised today that the 'grass-roots' expert may be literally on your doorstep. Better to ask the college kid next door to fix your laptop!

Living the Wisdom

Chances are, you have right now a big question in your life that needs an answer sometime soon. It might be whether to move house or whether little Jimmy should change schools. Whatever it is, if it's exercising your mind, expand the circle; trust some friends with it. Have them help you discuss the whys and the wherefores. And, if this kind of disclosure is already your practice, try discussing the issues with someone who you don't normally turn to in order to get a fresh perspective.

In summary, being open to fresh blood brings Young Brains more acquaintances, deeper friendships, more immediacy, fuller emotions, more unusual experiences, more trustworthy information, more ability to influence trends and better reasons to decide. That far-from-exhaustive list is already encouraging enough. Be informal, be open, be trusting and discover the benefits of fresh blood.

Young Brains remind us about the joys of friendship. When we were young we probably found making friends easy and instinctive – just like the Russian twins at the opening of the chapter. Subsequently, many of us have lost this Wisdom of Youth. Get it back by following a Young Brain mindset. Connect, belong and trust! Learn these lessons and be open to those whom you encounter on life's pathway.

Young Brain opportunities present themselves all the time but, if you've closed more doors than you should have closed, adjusting to new values and ways of thinking can be challenging. But it can also be a lot of fun. So aim for a point where meeting fresh blood is 'just what you like doing' and get on with it. Procrastination is one of the comfort zones of the Old Brain. Don't put it off. Start relating today.

SUMMARY OF GOALS

- Connect to new friends, especially draw from different backgrounds and ages: be informal and approachable.
- Harness the power of new technologies to create a friendship ecosystem.
- Seek out crowds: feel the emotion and make new contacts.
- Build trust by opening up to others.

Time to move on to the next Wisdom of Youth.

06

Being Always On

David couldn't believe how alive he felt. He was buzzing.

Eighteen months earlier he'd been laid low by a difficult divorce. His wife Suzie, who bubbled with energy and fun, had left him for another man, taking with her the two children he adored. The trauma had been deeply wounding. But from this distance he could see what had gone wrong.

She had been so full of energy, always wanting to go out and do things, see things and visit friends. He, on the other hand, had just wanted to spend evenings and weekends recovering from his demanding job. It had become a gnawing issue between them. As it went on, she seemed to get more energy, and he seemed to get less. Resisting her enthusiasm to go out and do things had drained him further.

Six months ago he had changed jobs, found a new flat and his life had taken off. Somehow an energy spring within him had been released. He was passionate about his work, excited by the things he got involved in away from his job, and was full of fun and activity with the kids when he got to see them.

If only he could have had access to this surge of energy two years earlier.

Defining being always on

Being always on is about being engaged in life and embracing its opportunities – and challenges – with infectious enthusiasm. It's about getting every ounce of pleasure and satisfaction out of your existence by being involved and excited about what is happening. Things, people, events, jobs, pastimes can all be interesting and involving if you decide not to sleepwalk through life. Of course, the choice is yours, but imagine what life could be like if you chose to squeeze every ounce of pleasure, satisfaction and reward out of it! So, why not 'burst Joy's grape' against your palate, in the words of the poet John Keats?

Young Brains understand and rise to the challenge. They want to get on with things. Now. They are up for it, whatever it is. No hanging about until they feel in the mood – just do something about the situation in hand. You never know when the phone will ring and you'll be invited to something that very evening – or when the boss will pop his head around the door to ask you urgently to attend an unexpected, high-pressured meeting. Equally, the chance to play a role in a future fundraising event or join a group of Sunday-morning cyclists may never come around again.

Let's face it, many people go around in a half-asleep dream world. A mundane and routine workaday life has reduced their levels of alertness and numbed their ability to react. When the chance comes, they miss it because they are simply not awake enough to take action. It's the serendipity thing – luck plus readiness means good and interesting things will probably happen.

'If it be not now, yet it will come: the readiness is all.'

Hamlet, Act V, William Shakespeare

The action taken may by impetuous – even foolhardy by Old Brain standards – but, as General Patton, the US general, pointed out towards the latter stages of the Second World War, a poor plan violently executed is a whole lot better than a perfect plan executed without vigour.

Violently executing plans – and sometimes taking vigorous action without a plan – is what youth does best. Energy and decisiveness are attractive aspects, which youth and Young Brains share: both engage and act.

'If the spirit doesn't move you, sit down and move your spirit.'

David Schwartz, *The Magic of Thinking Big*

Multitasking

How can you tell when someone is continually 'on'? He or she is opportunistic, actively listens to what you are saying, makes intelligent comments based on sound thinking, stays with things right to the end.

Being always on also means multitasking. If you are conscious and active, you can find yourself being hyperactive. Is it possible to phone someone whilst making the toast, feeding the baby in the highchair, with an eye on morning TV? Sure! Young Brains are multitaskers par excellence. Anything else is just wasting time.

Of course, Young Brains can sometimes be a positive danger to themselves and others with their enthusiasm for action. Driving while phoning hands-free and keeping an eye on the kids fighting in the back all the while listening to the GPS instructions is NOT to be recommended – but it's what Young Brains do anyhow. Young Brains reason that life is short, time is scarce and multitasking is a valid way of packing it all in.

For Young Brains, even their leisure life becomes a timed activity. How to maximise the evening ahead? Is it possible to go from work to the bar via the minimarket and then on to the bowling alley – and perhaps popping in at mum's house en route?

In Seville there is a superb oasis of peace, tranquility and shade in the heart of the dusty, hot city centre – the Jardines Reales Alcazares. In the calm serenity of the garden, sheltering under the cool shade of an orange tree against the roasting Andalusian sun, a young couple hustled into view and were heard saying: 'Come on, we've been here 20 minutes already and we planned to be at the Giralda bell tower for 1.30.' This may not strike you as the most commendable feature of a Young Brain, but being always on means they do not miss a trick – and see everything there is to see on their sightseeing trip to Seville.

An eagerness to get on with things is also demonstrable through another tactic the Young Brain uses to handle time. Predictably, an always on approach is extremely taxing and even the Young Brain needs to recuperate at some stage. How does it do this? In true intense fashion, of course. In this case, it means going as far and fast as possible and, until just before burnout, sleeping almost all weekend.

This is a kind of 'detox' attitude to poly-chronic life. Live full-on and then 'cure' yourself for a few days before going back to an action-filled life. To some readers, this may sound like madness, but it is perfectly rational to a Young Brain. For them, the greater madness is to spend your whole life with one foot on the accelerator and the other on the brake. How can you get anything done, when you are purposely holding yourself back?

Savouring your time

But being always on is also a broader and more complex concept than merely running around like a mad thing until your body screams at you to stop. It involves the thoughtful ability to change pace from time to time, which ties it entirely to the Wisdom of Youth, rather than the madness of youth.

Savouring your time is a crucial aspect of being always on, although at first sight it appears contradictory. The logic is that by savouring your time, you are left with greater space in your life for spontaneous things to happen. And plugging into spontaneous happenings is an important benefit of being always on in the widest sense.

The key element is that you need to be always on in an intelligent and measured way. If you are running at top speed, without being sensitive to what is going on around you, you won't notice the neighbour in the supermarket, the interesting article in the magazine, or the poster advertising 50 per cent off. Without down-time, you have no window in your diary to see an old friend who is in town, or to take up the offer of late tickets to a concert. On the other hand, if you have created time, you can stop to share a joke, have a chat and indulge in some horseplay.

Remember, even time planners tell you that you cannot 'fit' people into a precise timetable. The time you spend with others, if it is to be really meaningful to both parties, can never be finely judged or precisely allocated in advance.

So savouring your time is important. It involves the judicious and wise use of time, so that your energy can be deployed more effectively, and produce more enjoyment and satisfaction.

And, if you still think we are being paradoxical, that is probably because we are! Another thing Young Brains have assimilated is that the world is not often a linear, logical place. As they don't expect it to be, they are far more inclined to accept complexity, paradox and even disorder as a more usual state of things.

The message, then, is that it's increasingly okay to be paradoxical. It is entirely possible to engage in *gentle* physical exercise; or to play the *adagio* of a violin concerto at 100 decibels; or to go on *safe* adventure holidays. Equally, it is Young Brained to want to go fast in order also to go slow and vice versa.

Being in the flow

'Flow is about being completely involved in an activity for its own sake. The ego falls away. Time flies. Every action, movement, and thought follows inevitably from the previous one, like playing jazz. Your whole being is involved, and you're using your skills to the utmost.'

Mihaly Csikszentmihaly, *Flow*

Immersion in the moment – being in the flow – is another aspect of the Young Brain's ability to be always on. 'Flow' means being able to be completely focused and lost in whatever you are doing at a particular moment in time. It's about providing fruitful engagement and full satisfaction, rather than simply cramming everything in.

Remember how it feels to be so deeply immersed in your favourite hobby or pastime that you completely lose track of time? That's flow. And Young Brains know all about flow – and they know how to access it on a daily basis. As a consequence they live an intense, multicoloured, multi-sensory life. They are involved in their lives as active participants, not casual observers. Being always on means experiencing the true power of now.

Being always on, then, is about managing time intelligently. Sometimes it's right to fill every waking moment – as with the couple in Seville – and at other times it is most rewarding to savour some deep peace. On still other occasions, the most satisfying approach is to get totally absorbed in a task and, consequently, lose all track of time. The Wisdom of Youth is that, by having a flexible or polychronic approach to your time on earth, you create a life which is richer, more intense, more varied and, yes, younger!

Generating energy

Youthful get-up-and-go is about having energy to burn. It means never having to rein back your energy output in order to 'save a bit for later in the day'. And it means that the afternoon nap is an, as yet, untested concept.

Statistics clearly show that we lose – very rapidly – our (perceived) ability to access energy as we age. The fall-off in energy is dramatic from our teens onwards.

I feel full of energy

	15–17	18–24	25–34	35–44	45–54	55–64	65+
% Agree	63	53	43	37	33	29	21

Source: Sociovision 3SC UK, 2005

But diminishing energy levels are not predetermined by the ageing process. Just as some older people have bubbly irrepressible energy, we can all point to at least one teenager we know who gets up at noon, lazes around the house and barely has the energy to reply to a question with more than a grunt.

The important point to take away from the figures above is that over a third of 35–44-year-olds and a fifth of people over 65 *are* full of energy, so, whatever age category you fit into, you can be one of those who are still buzzing.

So while it is true that surplus energy is more natural in the young, to a large extent your energy levels are a state of mind.

Old Brains give themselves the licence to gently wind down their energy levels. Young Brains refuse to give in to apathy and general laziness. You can be energetic regardless of age, if you determine that this is what you want.

For example, the Young Brain can feel exhausted and yet can

transform its energy levels by controlling mind over body. Instead of flaking out, it goes to that evening event it was tempted to pass up on. Once there, new stimuli give it fresh energy to keep going enthusiastically into the early hours.

Irish multimillionaire Bill Cullen is well into his sixties. He is a firm believer in staying young, saying he never intends to retire. In his inspirational book, *Golden Apples*, he reveres Japanese physical fitness centres for the over-eighties – you have to be over 80 to join!

His book details his exercise, fitness and dietary philosophy, and is a model of its kind. Bill Cullen is definitely a Young Brain in an old body. He believes, for example, that sleeping is a waste of time. 'Sleeping is the nearest thing to dying you'll ever do, so don't do too much of it.' And the key to sleeping less – more physical exercise and more energy. As he also says: 'it's better to wear out than to rust out.'

Bill Cullen is planning ahead and wants to do more over the next 40 years than over his first 60. How will he do this? By continuing to have a Young Brain. 'Youth is inside you,' he says, 'it's your mental attitude and it's you who decides whether you are old or young. So make up your mind now that you can stay young by getting some projects to keep you busy.'

Bill Cullen, *Golden Apples*

Of course, everyone must judge for themselves just how much sleep they need – or can get away with. Certainly, medical science emphasises the value of sleep and we are definitely not suggesting sleep deprivation as a way to stay young! However, some of us actually require less sleep than we have convinced ourselves that we need. So it is well worth experimenting on what your body/mind requires at this juncture in your life. Remember, just 15 minutes less sleep per day adds up to 105 minutes a week or 7.5 hours per month. You could be always on for an extra 3.75 days a year if you found you could do without just a quarter of an hour's sleep per day!

It may seem like another paradox but, in order to gain more energy, you first need to use up what you've got on a regular basis. Think of top sportspeople. In order to be able to access high levels of energy when they perform competitively, they go through very rigorous daily training routines that take them to the point of exhaustion.

The same principle is true for us in our lives. The Wisdom of Youth says that it is a false economy trying to save energy by not expending it. Use it or lose it. Energy begets energy.

Young Brains access energy, Old Brains deny energy – it's as simple as that. David, in the story that opened this chapter, learned this the hard way.

We encounter here one of life's true virtuous circles. A sign of being youthful is the ability to expend energy. But, by so doing, adherents become fit and healthy and, here's the point, stay youthful longer. Turning towards action keeps Young Brains young.

Don't become lazy and fearful

'Men of age object too much, consult too long, adventure too little, repent too soon, and seldom drive business home to the full period, but content themselves with a mediocrity of success.'

Francis Bacon, 1561–1626

Can you be 'bothered'? Is getting dressed up and going out for an evening just too much hassle? Is speaking frankly to a superior just inviting trouble? Is regular exercise too tiring? If so, then there is a good chance you have an Old Brain.

You see, the Old Brain comes to be a lazy brain. Over time, it has grown comfortable, slow and flabby. And it has convinced itself that, while time may speed up as you age, your body inexorably slows down. What's more, there is nothing you can do about it.

So, it's another early night, another shunned opportunity.

Laziness is no more, and no less, a way of avoiding our fears. Life can be tough and the pain of living often leads us to retreat from life for fear of being hurt. Maybe you recognise this in some of your own actions? Most of us are prone to this failing.

During our lifetime, we inevitably have to endure physical suffering such as pain, sickness, injury, tiredness, and, eventually, death. And sometimes we have to endure psychological suffering such as sadness, fear, frustration, disappointment and depression. Indeed, one of Buddhism's Four Noble Truths is that 'life means suffering'.

Unless you have lived a very charmed life, chances are you have also suffered and maybe are currently going through difficult times.

Faced with such challenges, isn't it so much simpler just to duck facing up to them, or to contain problems by closing down responsiveness and reactivity to life in general? You feel the fear, but *don't* do it anyway. You end up in a rictus of doubt and inaction. You hope someone else will sort it for you (perhaps your partner will sort out the utility company which is coming after you – wrongly – for unpaid bills). You leave it to others to recycle and live sustainably (your efforts will be too small to make a difference anyway). You put off taking exercise (what difference will another day make?).

So, laziness and fearfulness go hand in hand. Out of fear of living, the Old Brain withdraws and becomes lazy by default. Being always on demands courage. And so does life. If you take the soft option, you'll be worse off in the end.

By adopting a 'safety first' strategy, the Old Brain condemns itself to a slow and fearful death, thus realising what it was seeking to avoid. The Wisdom of Youth, by contrast, says that the only way to stay young is to put fear behind you, be bold and throw yourself 100 per cent into your life.

The Young Brain has the courage to say: I'm not really sure where this is heading or what problems I'll encounter en route, but I'm in for the ride. Let's go for it. Harness this attitude in your own life and you will reap great benefits.

Benefits of being always on

The benefits are worthwhile and not to be missed:

- Keeping yourself fit and healthy.
- Strengthening your engagement to those closest to you.
- Maximising your time on earth; having no regrets.
- Being in tune with yourself, your feelings.
- Being open to luck and serendipity.
- Giving back; making a difference to the less fortunate.
- Having a more adventurous and interesting life.
- Becoming who you dream to be; having in your life what you desire to have.
- Holding your head high as you deal with life's challenges.
- Negotiating better deals.
- Making the most of new technologies and innovations.
- Experiencing new things, places and people.
- Surviving and flourishing in a competitive world.
- Compromising less.
- Making full use of your reserves of energy.

Adopt three Always-On mindsets as your own

As with the other five wisdoms, the benefits are so important that putting in the work to achieve a being always on mindset looks like a no-brainer. So what sort of thought patterns do Young Brains deploy in order to make sure they are always on? The three core ones are:

1 Learning by Doing

2 Searching for Mobility

3 Being Fearless (and having courage).

1 Some Learning by Doing Challenges

1 Are you the sort of person who cooks microwave meals and eats ready-made food? Or do you frequently get out the ingredients and make a meal?

2 The brakes on your bike aren't working properly: are you prepared to sort them out yourself?

If you are willing to get stuck in and get your hands dirty, you have a Young Brain mindset.

Be hands-on

People who are eager for action, ensure that life is much more than just an intellectual challenge. Okay, what goes on inside someone's head is extremely important and we've already said that a Young Brain needs to think itself young. But a Young Brain's wisdom also says that learning by doing is very important too. Being an impractical intellectual is a road to an ineffectual life. Being young at heart means rolling your sleeves up and getting dirty. Everything man-made we see around us is a *manifestation* of someone's thoughts. Wouldn't you rather make a tangible contribution to progress?

We mentioned before how Young Brains can be intuitive and often prefer to play with, say, a new technological device, rather than read the fine print of an instruction manual. This illustrates what we mean by learning by doing. Other examples include: a Young Brain would rather test drive a new car than spend time questioning the salesperson; a Young Brain cooks with a pinch of this, a dollop of that and a drizzle of the other rather than bother with the precision of a recipe; a Young Brain mostly prefers to explore a new city by wandering its streets rather than following in the footsteps of a tour guide.

In all three cases, the results may not always be optimal, but that is an acceptable compromise to the Young Brain, which ensures, at least, that he or she gets on with it. In any case, what is the alternative, asks the Young Brain? To take a salesperson's word for it? To spend so long mulling over a recipe book that dinner is late? To miss seeing the spontaneity and authenticity of local backstreet life in favour of a musty and dusty museum?

Leading celebrity chef Jamie Oliver is a Young Brained guy whose popularity stems from his informal 'learning by doing' cookery techniques. As anyone who has seen his TV shows, or read his books knows, he cooks with flair, instinct and cheekiness. He is completely hands on. Food, for him, is about getting his hands into the ingredients, 'ripping up bread, licking his fingers and getting a little tipsy'. It's about passing the parsnips and 'hanging out with friends and family'. His whole philosophy is to avoid being 'cheffy' whilst inspiring normal people to eat wholesome, flavoursome food, and all the while using shortcuts and tips to do it.

Living the Wisdom

DO things. Ideas you've mulled over to reorganise your life? Start making them happen. Seeing too little of your family? Hold a get-together. Your home environment needs revamping? Mend that chair and sort out the desk. Be brave, experimental and persistent.

Feel the pain

Recognise that taking an experiential approach can often be quite uncomfortable physically – but Young Brains do it anyway. For example, any reader who has hitch-hiked will know that getting around the country by this means allows you to meet all sorts of interesting people – and can be a huge learning experience. But end up at a motorway interchange after nightfall with rain running down your neck poses doubts even in the minds of the most resolute.

Trekking in Nepal is a wonderful learning experience, as anyone who has done it can testify, but are there moments of discomfort? You bet. Have you run a marathon? Did you hit 'the wall'? Running over 26 miles will test your endurance and your resolve; it will give you a new insight into your personal capacities and your physical perseverance, but it will also hurt – and hurt a lot. Learning by doing is often not for the faint-hearted – but Nike captured the spirit of this in their 'Just Do It' advertising campaign; pain is also the path that leads to glory – and youth.

Living the Wisdom

The next time you get a chance to take part in a charity hike, run or bike ride, go for it and relish the blisters – and the chance it gives you to learn more about yourself.

2 Searching for mobility

Mobility challenges:

1 Given the choice, would you take your vacation close to your home country or would you rather seek out foreign lands?

2 Do you prefer a quiet evening in or a night out on the town?

Explore your boundaries

Another mindset to adopt as you aim to be Always On is to search for mobility. Inaction roots you to the spot. You are stuck where you are. By contrast, action engenders movement.

Young Brains love to travel, discover and explore the world around them. Action to them can mean going to the cinema in the evening, potholing at the weekend or taking a year out to tour the world. But wherever 'it' is and for however long 'it' takes, it's all about actively getting out and about. Down with couch potatoes! Young Brains are on the move.

Perhaps the most thoughtful recent book on the nature of travelling was penned by Alain de Botton. This comment indicates succinctly what de Botton thinks travel tells us about our brains: 'If our lives are dominated by a search for happiness, then perhaps few activities reveal as much about the dynamics of this quest – in all its ardour and paradoxes – than our travels. They express, however inarticulately, an understanding of what life might be about, outside the constraints of work and the struggle for survival.'

Alain de Botton, *The Art of Travel*, 2002

Where have you travelled recently? What does this tell you about the nature of your brain and the constraints you place on your possibilities for action? What do your recent destinations reveal about your ambitions of what your life could be about?

Living the Wisdom

Get moving. Visit your local places of interest (you probably last saw them when you showed a nephew five years ago). If you can afford it, take weekend breaks in interesting locations. If you can't, find interesting places closer to home you could visit on a day's bike ride. And for that next holiday, try somewhere radically different.

Getting out

As you've seen, we are not only referring to long-distance travel. Being active and getting out and about can be as much about strolling to the shops or taking a picnic to the park. For we now live in a world where home life is being replaced by outdoor living. Think about it. Twenty years ago, if you wanted a coffee you'd go to your kitchen cupboard. Today you are just as likely to head for your nearest Starbucks or local equivalent.

And when you wanted a meal, this used to be something rustled up in the comfort of your home – not something you went out for – either sit-down or take away. And when you did go out into the wider world, it was with something very intentional in mind. 'I'm going to the shops.' 'I need to return the library books.' 'I've been invited for drinks in the neighbours' garden.' Very intentional and very much 'go out and come back as soon as it's finished'.

Today, home is just one of many options as a place for doing things. People are all out and about so much, we do things on the way to other outdoor activities. We no longer go out to shop, we shop when we are out.

Marketers call this being part of the new 'experience economy' – and many of us are hooked into it today. But it is the Young Brains who are most plugged in to this out-of-home existence. They are the 'see and be seen' group. Why would you want your home to be your castle, when you can go to the exciting new Thai restaurant, the uplifting yoga class or the sociable pub garden?

Some cultures are more oriented to an outdoor lifestyle than others. But the Australian culture is supreme in linking outdoor living with a zestful get-up-and-go mentality and a taste for spontaneity. In Europe, people tend to book social events into their diaries weeks in advance. Australians seem able to have nothing planned for that evening and then a magic ring-round process occurs. In no time, a beach party, BBQ or night on the town has been organised involving a group of 30 mates. Young Brains operate in the same manner – helped immeasurably, these days, by the ubiquitous text messaging. Want a party at the drop of the hat? Ask a Young Brain to organise it.

Opportunities in the new lifestyle economy now abound; the 'offer' has never been wider – but, to exploit all that is proposed, you have to take some action. Does it require energy to go clothes shopping? Absolutely. How much umph do you need to meet friends for a walk in the countryside? Bundles. Is it peaceful to take children or grandchildren camping? Not on your life! Living outside and exploiting the wider world requires immense reservoirs of energy, a real eagerness for mobility and a philosophy of being always on. Sitting at home with your slippers on and the newspaper in hand does not. It's as simple as that.

Living the Wisdom

Set a night a week aside for new activities – say Friday. Make it your mission to find some new experience for every Friday – for you, your partner, your friends or your family. Look on the Internet or in the local 'what's on'. You'll be amazed at the possibilities as you choose between 'bat watching', 'star gazing' or the 'local pub's quiz night' for next Friday's event.

3 Being fearless (and having courage)

Being fearless challenges

1 Do your fears stop you from engaging in new projects?

2 Do you feel deep down that, when the time is right, you are capable of making radical changes in your life?

Do success

It's a strange thing about human nature but, frequently, when people are on the verge of success and achieving their goals, they manage to shoot themselves in the foot. It's as if some of us have inner scripts which prevent us from being everything we could be.

Perhaps it's that little Old Brain voice inside our heads whispering negative thoughts: 'I am not worthy of this'; 'I don't deserve to succeed'; 'what will happen when people discover that I am only me?'

Psychologists working with leaders in business and other walks of life have identified something they call Impostor Syndrome. Impostor Syndrome often affects leaders when they are starting out, and sometimes creeps up on them even when they are experienced and successful. It defines the feeling that leaders get when they let fears and doubt creep in. They start wondering when they will be found out – surely any minute now, someone will spot they are not really a leader.

We all have these feelings from time to time, so, if you do too, don't worry, it's only human. It just means that to get the most out of life you need to have the courage to overcome these doubts.

> Some German ladies were talking in a focus group recently and one admitted to the others: 'I've achieved everything I ever dreamt about. I've got an adorable husband . . . two attractive, healthy kids . . we own our own apartment . . we go on exotic holidays. But, now that I've got all of this, it's as if I'm standing in my own way. I somehow prevent myself from being happy.'

Surely, stopping short of success is about fearing what will happen if one is successful. Putting your head above the parapet means taking a risk. Life may be changed for ever.

'Destroy fear through action.'

David Schwartz, *The Magic of Thinking Big*

The Wisdom of Youth is to feel this fear and do it anyway. Action overcomes our personal misgivings, our own tendency to self-destruct. Action pushes inertia to one side and allows Young Brains to triumph.

Living the Wisdom

The next time you feel uncertainty and doubt about a challenge, remind yourself you are not an impostor. You are a person who takes action, and is successful in that action. So battle on till your project is highly visible and successful. And keep the success going.

Act now, act radically

Plato said: 'The beginning is the most important part of any work.' A journey around the world starts with the very first step. The message is clear. Don't let procrastination thwart your plans, your dreams or your goals. Start acting today!

Young people are able to make the necessary changes to the way they live their lives to triumph against fear-induced inertia (see the following table). Being able to take radical action concerning who you are and how you live is an effective strategy to avoid the trap of complacency and hubris.

Sometimes I can decide very quickly to make radical changes in my life

	15–17	18–24	25–34	35–44	45–54	55–64	65+
% Agree	81	73	71	69	67	70	58

Source: Sociovision 3SC UK, 2005

Making such radical changes comes less easily once you're past you seventeenth birthday. However, blindly accepting the status quo 'we've always done it this way', is a quick way to atrophy and death.

And it's not only themselves that Young Brains dare to change. By tilting at windmills, Young Brains also perform a useful service to broader society. Can anyone forget the pictures of the young French students taking on the elite riot troops in the riots of 1968? Or the young Chinese student taking on the tanks in Tiananmen Square? Young people's fearlessness in pushing forward social and political frontiers can sometimes be breath-taking.

Living the Wisdom

If you need some better perspective concerning a big change you are contemplating, read Po Bronson's book, *What Should I Do With My Life?* This features more than 50 testimonies of people who've acted radically by changing their life's direction.

Take your courage in both hands

Young Brains are not merely fearless, they are also courageous. There is a difference. Since fear is often the anticipation of a future danger, fearlessness may be the result of pure ignorance of the risks or dangers involved.

Meanwhile, courage is about being brave when you are fully aware of what is going on, the adrenalin isn't pumping, and the natural thing to do is to slink quietly away and hide. This is particularly the case in the situations in which most of us are likely to find ourselves. The courage we need is not usually of the 'over-the-top-and-face-the-machine-guns' type, but the strength of character to make things happen in a hostile situation where vested interests are trying to keep things the way they are.

So Young Brains, are more likely to exhibit courage than fearlessness. This is decidedly more challenging. The person with a few years in the tank knows what can go wrong. And how much it can hurt.

Courage comes in many forms – physical, moral, intellectual or spiritual. There is a direct correlation between the amount of fear we feel, and the amount of strength of character we need to summon up to overcome that fear. We are talking here about the fundamentals of character. We need to stand for something – and accept the risks involved in going against the flow of popular opinion. We can't just have honour, dignity and self-respect in private. We may have to assert them in public, under adverse circumstances.

Being always on forces Young Brains to put themselves to the test in the glare of full publicity and have their integrity inspected at close quarters.

If you feel yourself some way from this sort of courage at the moment – don't worry. You may have been through a traumatic experience recently which has left you feeling vulnerable and lacking in assertiveness. We all go through difficult times when being courageous is especially challenging. However, we can assure you that you do have courage deep inside you that just needs teasing out and encouraging to reassert itself. There is no better time than the present to begin to rebuild your confidence by taking your courage in both hands.

Living the Wisdom

Get into the habit of being ready to stand up and be counted. Take a stand on an issue that is dear to your heart but one where you know you'll receive resistance from others. Get into a positive frame of mind by smiling as you enter the fray, and be sure not to get defensive or take resistance personally. Have the courage to argue your point and see it through. Be always on, and feel good about mixing it with the best!

SUMMARY OF GOALS

The great thing about being always on is that things get done. You feel good about yourself because something has been accomplished.

Young Brains have energy, drive, mobility and courage. Harnessing these strengths will help you to get going on the other Wisdoms of Youth.

- Stop sleep-walking through your life; it is not a dress rehearsal.
- Act your way to solutions rather than thinking your way through to answers.
- Get a life; get out and about.
- Do a scary thing every day and welcome success when it comes.

Now for the next Wisdom.

07

Hedonistic High

It was a hot, dusty Sunday afternoon in Coleman, Texas. It was high summer, 104 degrees, the fan was whirring over head and there was cool lemonade to be drunk.

Suddenly Jerry's father-in-law said, 'Let's get in the car and go to Abilene and have dinner in the cafeteria.' Jerry's first thought was 'Oh no. Fifty-three miles in high temperatures, a dust storm and no air-conditioning in the car.' Before he could open his mouth, his wife had chimed in saying what a great idea it was. To keep the peace, Jerry also said it was a great idea, but doubted whether his wife's mother would want to go. Not to be left out, the mother enthused 'Of course I want to go.'

So off the four of them went in the brutal heat with dust penetrating every orifice of the car. Before long it was cemented onto their bodies by their sweat. The food at the cafeteria was awful and, by the time they had completed the round trip, no one was speaking.

Once back, the family sat on the veranda in silence. Jerry eventually broke it by saying, 'It was a great trip, wasn't it?' More silence. It was left to his mother-in-law to speak up: 'Well, to tell the truth, I really didn't enjoy it much and would much rather have stayed here. I wouldn't have gone if you hadn't all pressured me into it.'

Everyone else exploded in turn. It was a crazy idea, no one had wanted to go, they had all felt blackmailed into going. In the words of Jerry, 'After the outburst of recrimination we all sat back in silence. Here we were, four reasonably sensible people who, of our own volition, had just taken a 106-mile trip across a god-forsaken desert in a furnace-like temperature through a cloud-like dust storm to eat unpalatable food at a hole-in-the-wall cafeteria in Abilene, when none of us had really wanted to go. In fact, to be more accurate, we'd done just the opposite of what we wanted to do. The whole situation simply didn't make sense.'

Defining hedonistic high

We've all done it. It's what management scientists such as Jerry B. Harvey – the hero of the tale – call the inability to manage agreement. The subtext, of course, is the inability to manage disagreement. In other words, the desire to avoid conflict. Old Brains aren't comfortable with conflict, as it takes them well outside what they are comfortable with. Conflict may lead to rejection. And rejection may lead to separation, alienation and loneliness. Don't risk it, counsels the Old Brain.

This is a paradox – the Abilene paradox. It's our fear of taking risks that may, ultimately, result in our separation from others – especially people whom we love. The irony is that, in not speaking up, we find ourselves separated anyway, because we don't agree with what is going on or the decisions that have been made.

Irony upon irony, it takes a whole lot of teamwork to get to Abilene. People give up their comfort and peace of mind to go there. And, in colluding with others to get there, we further reduce our capacity to be spontaneous and say what we think.

Young Brains are less contaminated with the desire to please at all costs. They are more spontaneous and fearless, and call a spade a spade. They refuse to sacrifice their own pleasure and satisfaction on the altar of consensus and political correctness. Their natural spontaneity and honesty avoids the self-defeating nature of the Abilene paradox. They follow their urges and decide what option will give them the greatest happiness.

You know that feeling you have when you sit watching a TV programme that you don't want to watch but, in a moment of weakness, agreed to? Maybe it's yet another boring football match – or charmless reality TV. The sentiment is not only one of frustration at having given in but also of a pleasure denied.

You could have been watching that film you know you would have loved. Or better still, reading a book.

The problem is that some people go through their whole lives with this dull ache inside. Somehow, they are not getting the same amount of happiness out of life that others seem to be getting. It's as if their entire existence was being spent watching the metaphorically wrong TV channel. The compromises they make, the consensus they seek, doesn't leave any room for their own pleasure. They are missing the hedonistic high.

Young Brains, by contrast, are more in tune with their basic needs. It's as if they have a hotline directly to the pleasure zone in their brain and this dictates their decisions and actions. Accordingly, they take positive measures to ensure that the life they live is full of happiness and spontaneous laughter. This is what hitting the hedonistic high is all about. Tapping into that highway that leads directly to pleasure.

For example, Young Brains know immediately and instinctively what music to put on in order to suit their mood and give them maximum pleasure. Out of a whole lighting department, they are able to gravitate to the very lamp that gives them the biggest kick. In a delicatessen, they know instinctively the food they will find the most mouth-watering.

And here's the thing. It's not only that their choices give them the most personal pleasure, but that everyone around senses the judicious nature of their decisions too. You've perhaps had this experience. You are invited to dinner by a friend and, from the moment you walk in, to your departing goodbyes, everything is perfect – just as it should be. The music captures the mood, the lighting level is spot-on and the food combination sublime. The French call this 'l'art de vivre' and the skill is indeed the talent to live life to the full – to attain the hedonistic high.

The Wisdom of Youth says: aim for a hedonistic high in your life – and avoid that meaningless and uncomfortable trip across the desert.

Finding happiness

Young people experience more happiness in their lives. Life, it would seem though, becomes less entertaining as we age.

It's important I have a life full of entertainment and excitement

	15–17	18–24	25–34	35–44	45–54	55–64	65+
% Agree	87	85	78	76	67	67	58

Source: Sociovision 3SC UK, 2005

How much of this joylessness is a fact of life and how much is due to one's approach to life? Again, we suggest that life chances are largely influenced by one's attitude. Older people, and particularly Old Brains, tend to let emotional dullness and melancholy happen to them.

Young Brains, on the other hand, have an intense desire to find entertainment, joy and laughter wherever it is available. As we shall discover, they have developed the necessary mindsets to keep fun flowing in their lives.

One other point to make before we move on with our exploration of the hedonistic high. Avoiding the traps of the Abilene Paradox has some crossovers with enlightened selfishness, but it is a separate and distinct wisdom. Enlightened selfishness is essentially concerned with the inner you – it is introspective in that it relates to protecting yourself from shrivelling and creating opportunities to flower as a person. Hedonistic high, on the other hand, is outward-looking, and relates to a positive approach to being playful and creating opportunities for joy and happiness.

Don't be sad

Old Brains tend to live in a more or less permanent state of sense-of-humour failure.

Worry, stress, responsibilities, the daily grind have all conspired to take the fun out of life. It's a serious business, living. Stop smirking at the back.

The trouble is that Old Brains don't even consider smirking these days. They've forgotten what mischief is. They've lost the knack of fooling around. And when they see others being frivolous or playful, they find it all mildly embarrassing. It's the sort of thing young children do. But adults – of any age – not really!

In wartime Britain there was a popular radio programme featuring the comedian Tommy Handley, which kept both civilians and troops laughing. One of Tommy's characters was Mrs Moanalot, who, with her non-stop moaning, well and truly lived up to her name. Her catchphrase was 'Aye. It's being so cheerful that keeps me going.'

One of the core reasons that Old Brains aren't cheerful is that, like Mrs Moanalot, they often have little insight into themselves and their own oddities. Their sense of humour failure stems from an inability to laugh at themselves. They tend to be rigidly defensive, and entrench themselves behind the barricades of position and status. Laughing takes them out of their comfort zone; it entails risk and loss of status. This makes them prickly and po-faced.

Young Brains, of course, find it entirely natural to laugh at themselves. The human race is essentially absurd, and Young Brains are sufficiently self-knowing to recognise the fact. For example, a Young Brain was talking recently about a dinner party she hosted where the main course, a quiche, burned badly in the oven. She served it to her guests, nevertheless, with the humorous instruction to simply strip off the black crust since it was perfect underneath!

In the same situation an Old Brain would be sent spinning. A burned quiche would have been treated as a serious faux pas. There would have been red faces, profuse apologies to the guests, a frantic scrabbling around to serve something else entirely. Possibly, even begging for forgiveness and then expiating his guilt by committing 'hari kiri'.

Monty Python mercilessly sent up traditional ways of thinking. Many sketches were woven around the stubborn mentality of Old Brains ('This Norwegian Blue is not dead, it's just pining for the fjords.') You may also remember the sketch where a diner at a restaurant table complains that his knife is dirty. This leads to a series of unintended and hilarious consequences as members of staff, ever more senior, come to apologise for their grave error. The sketch ends with the French chef begging for forgiveness and then 'doing the honourable thing'.

Old Brains simply are not on the lookout for joyful, or delightful occasions or experiences and so find them a lot less often. Old Brains miss out on a lot of fun.

Maybe you can confirm this observation in your own life. There are people who simply cannot take any pleasure in receiving a gift. Yes. Even the idea of a present, given from the heart, is not enough to make this kind of person smile. He or she shrugs his or her shoulders, grimaces or even criticises the gift or the giver ('You shouldn't have/I've got everything I need/It's too expensive'). What they singularly do not do is to grin and thank the giver with enthusiasm.

Or again, do you know parents who are so concerned with principles and the right upbringing, that even the most charming acts of their offspring are met with a scowl? A toddler arrives and proudly shows her muddy hands, having spent a happy moment in the garden, and all the parent can think of is giving a lesson in propriety and cleanliness. The same messy behaviour would be met by broad smiles and a snap for the photo frame by another parent. Which parent, in your opinion, has the older brain?

Ultimately, all this can add up to a fairly sad life. Lack of a happy disposition leads to negative interpretations of events. And a vicious circle can develop whereby negative events can lead to an even unhappier disposition.

Similarly, being sad only serves to attract friends who are equally despondent.

Contrast these Old Brain traps with the benefits of being on a hedonistic high.

Benefits of hedonistic high

- Saving time for what you really want to be doing in your life – avoiding trips to Abilene.
- Making lots of new, fun friends.
- Feeling the joy of getting other people laughing; sharing your happiness and spreading the glow.
- Leading life as an adventure.
- Opening yourself to being luckier.

- Beginning to feel you are blessed – one of life's happy few.

- Feeling alive and with lots of energy.

- Releasing yourself from meaningless rituals and senseless obligations.

- Relishing the joy of creating or participating in mischief.

- Reaping life's rewards for all the hard work you put in elsewhere; fun makes it all worthwhile.

- Feeling the joy and satisfaction of belonging to a family or close group who laugh together.

Adopt three Hedonistic High mindsets as your own

Once again, to help you harness the benefits of hedonistic high, we have identified three mindsets that Young Brains naturally adopt, enabling them to confront life with a twinkle in their eye and joy in their heart:

1 Seeking Pleasure

2 Laughing a Lot

3 Riding Luck.

1 Seeking pleasure

Pleasure challenges

1 If someone asked you if you would like to try quad biking, how would you answer?

2 You are asked to join a prestigious committee which you see as deadly boring? Do you accept?

So, do you need more Pleasure in your life?

Having fun

Young Brains, it has to be said, have a heightened desire to seek pleasure. They seem to instinctively understand that it is not only pleasant to have fun, it is also important. Having a laugh needs to be taken seriously. So, says the Young Brain, let's go out of our way to ensure fun comes our way. Let's take risks and be thrilled by life.

I enjoy taking risks – it's important I have an exciting life

	15–17	18–24	25–34	35–44	45–54	55–64	65+
% Agree	92	89	77	69	56	51	30

Source: Sociovision 3SC UK, 2005

The table above hardly needs comment. The very young go gung-ho for fun. By 25 life is a bit more serious, and the quest for excitement tumbles as soon as early adulthood and 'Old Brain' thinking starts to take root. By the time people are over 65, risk taking and excitement is much rarer in their lives.

The latter may believe things like fulfilment and contentment are pretty important – and they are – but that need not preclude a bit of over-the-top fun. Indeed, it could be said that mischief is a staple of a Young Brain. The capacity to be a bit subversive goes with the territory. Roald Dahl was in his sixties when he wrote *The Twits*, demonstrating that a Young Brain of any age can mix it with the best of them when it comes to fun and naughtiness.

'Mr Twit thought that his hairiness made him look terrifically wise and grand. But in truth he was neither of these things. Mr Twit was a twit. And now at the age of 60 he was bigger twit than ever.'

Roald Dahl, *The Twits*

Pleasure-seeking can take many forms but essentially has both softer and harder sides. Soft pleasure includes more discerning pursuits linked to art and culture. Having a good time at a museum, sampling good wines, having friends around are all soft pleasures. So is playing with your children or joking with an old acquaintance. Such simple pastimes give you a warm, fuzzy feeling and make it so much easier to see the funnier side of life.

Hard hedonisms are cruder and more thrill-seeking. These might include an extreme sport, a night out on the town or a rowdy time with your mates. It is also being obsessed with comic books and dressing up in superhero costumes, for example – or sweating through a full-on 'abs' workout. Whatever appeals! Unless things get too excessive or nasty, hard pleasure is an equal source of fun and laughter. Letting your hair down is a relief and a respite from life's stresses and has much to recommend it.

Avoid the unpleasant

You may be familiar with *Jackass*, the American TV series which has now spun off into two Hollywood movies. *Jackass* was shown originally on MTV and features people performing various dangerous, crude, ridiculous and self-injuring stunts and pranks. A more faithful rendition of what the hard hedonism urge is all about, you could not find.

Of course, Old Brains find all of this entirely distasteful, even corrupting. Sensible Young Brains might recognise the need for limits, but also see

Jackass as a simple extension of the 'video gag' shows where people, pets and property have unintended pratfalls, all filmed on amateur videos. Is it funny to see people slip on a banana skin? You bet! It always has been and always will be. We were made to laugh, so why hold it in?

Living the Wisdom

Try to light up your life. Over the coming weeks ensure that you have some fun – mischief or horseplay or preferably both. You may have to 'plan' this – like most comedians plan their routines – but don't let this worry you. The point is to have a laugh, not necessarily to be quick-witted.

Lighten things further by choosing to be surrounded by fun-loving friends and light-hearted leisure activities. For the near-term future, read mostly funny books and watch films that make you laugh.

Another obvious tactic when seeking pleasure, Young Brains find, is to avoid unpleasurable situations. Letting things go, leaving worries behind, not being dragged down by the world's woes, these are all legitimate ways of keeping the pecker up.

Above all, Young Brains understand that the world is divided up into 'Radiators' and 'Drains'. Radiators are the people who beam a warm glow of energy and joy. They are life-enhancing and a joy to be with. Drains, on the other hand, suck the life out of you. They are joyless and life-reducing. They are poisonous and to be avoided at all costs. Even if they are related to you or are a friend.

It is rare, but not unheard of, for Young Brains to change jobs several times in one year – just looking for the one where they can really have fun *during* the working day. In one specific case, a candidate for a job in a retail store was asked for his questions at the end of the recruitment interview. Reflecting for a moment about how his destiny could be in the balance, he paused and then asked: 'Do you have great parties?' This kind of attitude drives Middle-aged Brains mad: how is it possible to recruit someone whose main criterion is their personal fun-seeking? From a Young Brains' viewpoint, however, it is entirely logical that their performance will be predicated upon their state of mind and enjoyment of the job and the culture. A happy worker is a good worker.

Young Brains understand that it is important to avoid an unhappy career, as it's a route to emotional disaster. Young Brains refuse to mortgage current happiness; they refuse to live life only for tomorrow and tolerate an unhappy today.

Living the Wisdom

Be firm in your intention to change for the better. Select a Drain that gets you down whenever you see him or her, and decide on a plan to neutralise or cut them out your life. Harsh? Yes. Necessary? Absolutely.

Putting things into perspective

Pleasure-seeking is also an antidote to all the bad news in the world today. Doomsayers are flooding the market with the stark message: 'you ain't seen nothing yet'. Just look at the titles of some of the material released over the last few years. There's been Al Gore's *An Inconvenient Truth*; Stephen Leeb's *The Coming Economic Collapse*; Peter Navarro's *The Coming China Wars*; and Paul Robert's *The End of Oil*, to name but a few. James Martin's admirable *The Meaning of the 21st Century* begins with the lines: 'At the start of the 21st century, humankind finds itself on a non-sustainable course, a course that, unless changed, will lead to catastrophes of awesome consequences. This could be humanity's last century.'

Dire stuff. Now add in the World-wide recession and it's enough to make pessimists of all of us, or send the World into a morass of gloom and doom. Except that this very uncertain and threatening climate is one principal reason for the Young Brain's desire for spontaneity and laughter – even if the humour is sometimes very black. The Young Brain says, faced with this depressing context, let's make the most of our lives.

This was, remember, the very response of the golden generation of youth in the swinging Sixties. The Cold War, and with it a very genuinely felt sense of imminent nuclear destruction on a worldwide scale, produced both joy and the celebration of life on an epic scale. Irreverence, spontaneity and free sex were the watchwords, and The Beatles, The Rolling Stones and Bob Dylan ruled the World.

More recently, this was the surprising finding after New York's terrifying 9/11 cataclysm. Manhattan's bars and clubs were full in the subsequent weeks, contrary to all expectations. Rather than turning inward towards tradition, with a sense of seriousness and sobriety, Young Brains decided that, given life's fragility, the best tactic was to celebrate the fact they were alive and kicking.

Digging a little deeper, this behaviour is very revealing about the way the Young Brain works. It's not that Young Brains do not see the deep concerns in the collective sphere; nor is it that they don't care – they do, passionately. However, they are ready to separate what happens more broadly in society with what happens in their private sphere. For Young Brains, it is entirely possible to be depressed and disillusioned about the plight of the world and happy and confident in their own personal lives. 'Have fun while you can . . . for tomorrow we die' is the Young Brain's motto.

Living the Wisdom

Take a holiday from newspapers, TV, etc. for two weeks – they are Drains, and poisoners of all things positive. You'll be amazed at how much more positive and joyful the world is without them.

2 Laughing a lot

Laughing challenges

1 Do you have a good belly laugh on an almost daily basis?

2 Do you systematically delete emails from friends who send round batches of jokes or fun photos?

Laugh at yourself

Underpinning all humour is the ability to laugh at ourselves. This may be painful – if we are the butt of satire or some other form of send-up – but we lose this ability at our peril.

Most of the time Old Brains don't find themselves funny. Young Brains do.

Laughing at yourself is a great way to demonstrate that you don't take yourself too seriously. It shows you have enough self-confidence and self-regard not to worry about looking silly. Only people with fragile egos, debilitating insecurities or Old Brains fear laughing at themselves. Those with a healthy self-image relish the opportunity to connect with others through self-effacing humour. It demonstrates they have insight into themselves and their failings. It shows they have warmth and humanity.

Smile about the small stuff

Young Brains adopt a mindset which enables them to laugh at life. Whereas others simply miss the joke, Young Brains delight in finding the humorous side of life. Father Christmas loses his beard. That adds a lot more fun! There's no corkscrew in the picnic hamper. Who needs wine anyway – that water from the natural spring will do the trick. The wind blows the tent down. Great – free air conditioning!

If you have the right attitude, even life's little problems become a reason to laugh.

This is not a hard wisdom to learn, but how many of us react in the opposite way? Life goes wrong and we take it as further proof that everything is going against us. At the same time, we are jealous of the popular guy or girl at work who is surrounded by friends and always seems to see the funny side of life. Odd, that.

Spread some

Allied to being able to laugh a lot is the concept of spreading a little happiness. Maybe you caught the film *Amélie* with Audrey Tautou taking the starring role and playing a young lady who makes it her mission to bring light and laughter into the lives of her neighbours – and even strangers.

> During Jean-Pierre Jeunet's inspiring film, Amélie inadvertently discovers a rusty toy tin belonging to a former inhabitant of her flat. Seizing serendipity by the hand, Amélie takes the opportunity to bring some light into someone's life. She tracks down the owner, the toy is returned and her actions bring marvellous benefits. Determined in her new role as a 'facilitator' for other people's wellbeing, Amélie sets off helping blind people through town and creating harmony in the love lives of her café colleagues.

This uplifting film hits this particular mindset bang on the head. The idea is that by doing some little kindness, having a sunny disposition and laughing often, you will have a subtle, yet meaningful effect on everyone around you. Some would go even further and maintain that, by spreading some light-heartedness, a chain reaction forms and the whole world will smile.

While, for many Young Brains, the idea that a small action can have a huge impact is a simple act of faith, mathematicians have confirmed this belief in their work on the theory of chaos.

> Mathematicians talk about this as 'the sensitive dependence of initial conditions' – more popularly known as the 'butterfly effect'. The theory holds that small variations of the initial condition of a non-linear dynamical system may produce large variations in the long-term behaviour of the system. For example, a ball placed at the top of a hill may run into completely different valleys according to its precise initial placement.

So the butterfly effect supports the age-old saying: 'Laugh, and the world laughs with you.' As well as appreciating the galvanizing effect of joy and humour in everyday life, the Young Brain also understands the flip side of the coin: 'Cry, and you cry alone.'

Be happy to become happier

It is notable that happiness and joy are part of a self-fulfilling prophecy. In recent studies of happiness and wellbeing (an area of research now called 'happiness studies') psychologists and sociologists have used detailed surveys to explore and measure people's subjective assessments of their life satisfaction.

There is now a broad body of supporting evidence which suggests that people who rate their life satisfaction and happiness highly have been independently observed to smile and laugh more than those who score lower. In separate checks, respondents' friends have been consulted, and their views tend to tally very closely with the self-assessments. So they are not just putting on a brave face for the questioner.

While it may seem blindingly obvious to non-researchers, it's good to have it confirmed – if you have the capacity to enjoy life, and are grateful for what you've got, you are more likely to have a lot more laughs and smile more often as you pass on your merry way.

Further proof of this positive feedback comes from medical science. Serotonins are hormones released by the brain, and scientists believe them to play an important role in the regulation of anger, aggression, body temperature, mood, sleep, sexuality and appetite. Low levels of serotonin may be associated with several disorders, namely increase in aggressive and angry behaviours, clinical depression, obsessive-compulsive disorder (OCD), migraine, irritable bowel syndrome and anxiety disorders.

However, high levels of serotonin have the reverse effects and it is not for nothing that they have been termed the 'happy chappies' of our endocrine system. While genetic and environmental factors dictate your natural levels of serotonin, assuming you have a working level to start with, the important point is that happiness and laughter cause more serotonin to be released. It is literally true that laughing can make you mentally healthy.

Living the Wisdom

There is a moment when you are laughing or happy when you can almost feel the release of serotonin in your system. Try this. Say to yourself ten times, 'I am happy.' As you do so, smile and really mean it. Did you feel something, somewhere welling up inside you making you feel more positive? We hope so because that's the effect you are looking for. You may even find yourself smiling minutes later.

Focus hard on increasing your laugh and smile count each day (be serious about this, it's no laughing matter) and get those happy chappies circulating freely in your blood.

Fun and friendship

It goes without saying that fun and laughter are often conditioned by human relationships. It is therefore vital only to enter into friendships where you can relax, feel at ease and lighten up. As we mentioned earlier, avoid unpleasant people. This simple rule relieves you from a lifetime of vicious gossip, childish bickering and depressing negativity.

As we saw in an earlier chapter, seeking fresh blood can have numerous benefits. Here's another. If you have a wide circle of friends you may well be able to identify the young-brained fun-seekers among them. Having done so, you can then afford to take the 'wild side' with these individuals – and have a lot of fun in the process. Meanwhile, your broad circle of pals ensures that you are not risking your entire network by your hedonistic pursuits.

Living the Wisdom

Go through everyone you know – in your head or on paper – and mark those whose approach to life is unreservedly fun-loving. Hint: they are the ones who are always joking and who have very visible laughter lines around their eyes and mouths. Actively seek out these friends – and dodge the others.

---

3 Riding luck

Riding luck challenges

1 If someone offers you a hand when you need it, do you typically accept your good luck with open arms – or do you politely refuse his or her help?

2 Do you let the feeling of being unlucky weigh you down?

Look out for it

Let's turn to another way Young Brains ensure that they live a spontaneous and fun-filled life. By now you may have detected a certain undercurrent of spirituality in the Young Brain's mindset. This is not necessarily in the sense of being religious, but more about being open to happenings and influences that are beyond the dimension of the day to day. This siding with the inexplicable is very apparent when we talk about the riding luck mindset.

Luck is a very old-fashioned notion and we think about things like rabbits' feet and black cats. All cultures are embedded with tales and superstitions of what brings good luck, and what are the harbingers of bad luck. Young Brains take the principle of luck and add a self-determination twist: they say, luck plus the ability to take hold of luck by its horns is what is needed in modern life.

So when Lady Luck looks your way, be ready to make room for her.

What does riding luck mean in practical terms? When you are looking for a job move and the right post jumps off the vacancies page you were only vaguely scanning, that is serendipity at work. Follow this chance factor and make that application now. When you have a problem with your tax return and you just stumble upon a dinner guest who knows the answer, you need to take that good fortune and turn it to your advantage.

Or what about this? When your daughter is having problems with her maths and you happen upon exactly the book that can help her at your local jumble sale or car boot sale, you ride that luck. How about that moment when you are desperate for company and an old friend rings? Jump at the chance and invite them around. That, too, is serendipity in full flood.

It's a sad truth, but many people give up on luck. Are you one of those? Are you someone who will never buy a raffle ticket, scratch a lottery card or take a chance on a fairground stall? Despite your protestations, this may say nothing about your attitude to 'a little flutter' and a whole lot about your openness to good fortune.

Living the Wisdom

Take a good look at yourself and give yourself an honest answer to the questions: Do I believe I can be lucky? Do I believe I deserve to be lucky? If the answers are 'no' and 'no', then you must really work on becoming open to luck. You must start to look for it, accept it – and, finally, be grateful for it.

It's too easy. So what?

Chance encounters and lucky finds are so easily ignored. Older brains can get so hung up on the need to make a conscious effort in order to solve something, that even if the answer they need comes up and bites them on their backside, they will ignore it. If it is easily had, says the older brain, then it is probably worthless. We've got news for these people: diligence is not the only route to destiny.

Living the Wisdom

When serendipity looks sweetly upon you, say YES and kiss luck on the lips!

Luck and emotions

And being lucky can be a source of amusement as well as success. An amateur collector who scours junk shops and stumbles upon a rare art deco figurine can dine out on the story for months. Two strangers who meet by accident on a foreign holiday can end up sharing the rest of their vacation, and spend much of it giggling about their good fortune.

Riding luck is also about having no regrets. Seeing life as a giant roulette wheel, Young Brains are prepared to place bets and possibly get wiped out before starting again. For them, this is not losing but *learning*. Only by having regrets do you lose. Regrets only weigh you down and prevent future spontaneity.

How many Old Brains live lives of sadness and quiet desperation having lost a loved one? How is it possible to ride this savage bad luck? One clear response is to be grateful about what you had, feel no regrets, and then move on by opening yourself to spontaneous events and encounters. Easily said, of course, but a positive belief in the beneficence of Lady Luck definitely helps support the morale in life's challenging periods.

Living the Wisdom

When you have been lucky, say so and really enjoy the positive pleasures that come from a completely unexpected boon.

That was a lucky decision

We all face a multitude of decisions each day and they can weigh us down – especially the big ones. But a belief in luck and some sort of universal goodness can lighten our decision-making and help us get on the move. Young Brains accept this wisdom. They have faith that 'if you leap, the net will appear'.

How many times have you looked at the good fortune of others and said: 'Oh! They were just lucky. They were in the right place at the right time'? Putting any jealousy to one side, maybe you have put your finger on it, actually; they were lucky. But they were only lucky because they made their luck by being bold in their decision-making. In life, fortune really does favour the brave.

It happens when you decide to leave a bad job and find yourself later in exactly the area you dreamed about working in. It happens when you go off the beaten track on holiday and stumble across something simply stunning. It happens when you and your mates decide not to sit in on a rainy Sunday afternoon and the sun comes out and shines down on your hillside walk.

Living the Wisdom

Next time you have a decision to make, factor in a healthy dose of good luck. Have faith that the gods are looking down kindly on whatever course of action you finally decide on. Then get ready to let the good times roll.

SUMMARY OF GOALS

- Seek out pleasure; it's not sinful and will do you a great deal of good.
- Laugh at yourself and laugh with others, frequently.
- Trust to luck and be ready to go where it takes you.

Enjoying fun and laughter in the company of others really isn't that difficult – once you get back into the Young Brain way of reacting to life.

As the saying goes, 'Enjoy!'

08

Designing Tomorrow

In 1783, the American polymath Benjamin Franklin, was standing in the Parisian gardens of the rue de Montreuil, watching the first flight by man. Two intrepid adventurers were taking their lives in their hands in a balloon constructed by the Montgolfier brothers. Once they were airborne, a spectator turned to Franklin and asked, 'Sir, frankly, what is the use of flying in the air?' To which Franklin replied, 'Sir, what is the use of a newborn baby?'

Defining designing tomorrow

It has been said that the best way of predicting the future is to create it yourself. This is another way of saying that either you control your own life or life controls you. The Wisdom of Youth rejects the shrug-of-the-shoulders fatalism that accepts to be the victim of events. It says that the world is your oyster – so go and make something of it!

As we have stressed throughout this book, personally taking control of your life is even more important today than in the past. When the world spins slowly on its axis, going along with events is fine, and has the virtue of stability and predictability. Who wants to make waves when the tides of change shift slowly and caress you into peaceful slumber?

Fast forward to the present. The world is spinning much faster. Things happen more quickly, and you have to make a conscious effort to retain some sort of coherence and direction in your life.

Nobody really wants to be at the mercy of other people or world events – being tossed about by stormy seas is no fun; much better to design your own lifeboat. Today, more than ever, creating your own future is the only sensible response.

Young Brains have accepted responsibility for their future and eagerly pursue its creation.

For a start, they are highly imaginative and have a firm belief in the power of mental representation. In other words, they have developed the ability to see how they want things to be in their mind's eye. Sculpting their personal environment in an imaginative, thoughtful way, is one way of taming the world.

The problem is that we were all born with more imagination than we allow ourselves as adults to believe. Somehow, teaching methods and the grind of daily life have choked our visionary capacities. Yet again, we have lost the Wisdom of Youth.

Young Brains have ferociously hung on to their imagination, however. And they exercise imagination in all areas of life – not just the touchable/tangible. Careers are thought through and where they want to get to is visualised, long before they make it happen. Relationships, too, are projected out before they are played out. In their leisure lives, too, they use visualisation techniques, for example, to see themselves scoring the winning goal long before getting to the park and playing.

It all comes down to a desire to foresee the future and thereby shape it. If you can't predict where you might be heading, how do you know whether you are on the right road?

'Younger generations ... want to be in control of their lives ... want to extend their sense of authorship from how they design their living rooms to how they conduct their careers, to feel autonomous, take the initiative and be rewarded with a sense of achievement and recognition.'
Charles Leadbeater *We-think*

With imagination we can invent personal realms, unfold new life stories, create new narratives. And if we can first convince ourselves in our private world – we can then set out to convince others in the real world.

This may seem to run contrary to the propensity to go with the flow that we talked about earlier. In fact the paradox is easily resolved. Young Brains show a highly developed ability to discriminate between the elements in their life they judge to be strategic – which justify prefiguring and preplanning – and those less important aspects, where flow and serendipity can come into play.

This brings out another skill which Young Brains nurture: creativity. This is applied imagination. Creativity is the bridge between what you see in your mind's eye and what the world sees. It involves doing something fresh or original. To qualify as being creative, however, the outcome has to be recognised to have built some new value. That means it should alter the world in some way – or at least our perception of it. A 'creative output', by definition, shapes the world – and thereby helps a Young Brain to master his or her environment.

Once again, creativity is not sent as a gift from above but it is something that has to be practised. And, while it may have been more natural in childhood, Young Brains need to put in consistent work and maintain good habits to keep it fully functional and in order.

'There is a process that generates creativity – and you can learn it. And you can make it habitual. No one is born with that [creative] skill. It is developed through exercise, through repetition, through a blend of learning and reflection that's both painstaking and rewarding.'

Twyla Tharp, *The Creative Habit*

Of course, creativity includes endless possibilities. These could be writing a book, interpreting some music, painting a poster or designing a building. Or it might be running an organisation, or launching a business. On a more day-to-day level, it might be simply finding a new way to fold the ironing or trying new colours or types of garden plants.

While we are provoked by our context to be imaginative and creative, we are also fortunate to live at a time when the means to remake the world around us (political, artistic, domestic, technological ...) is available to almost everyone. The Wisdom of Youth is to acknowledge this and *design tomorrow*.

Tapping creativity

Employing our imagination and being creative is one of the most enjoyable aspects of rediscovering the Wisdom of Youth.

As our brains age, we tend to use our creativity and imagination less and less. The following table demonstrates this starkly. Once we hit 25, we start accepting the world as it is, rather than remaking it as we would like it to be. The fall-off is particularly strong after the age of 65.

I often create my own World, somewhere between reality and imagination

	15–17	18–24	25–34	35–44	45–54	55–64	65+
% Agree	57	61	54	45	47	44	32

Source: Sociovision 3SC UK, 2005

Part of youth's drive is to create new music, new art, new approaches, new ways of thinking – in fact, anything that brings something different and original to the party.

Young Brains think likewise. How else to explain the 70-year-old inventor in his garden shed, or the 50-year-old woman about to launch her new jewellery-making business?

There is no age limit to being creative: you just need to rejuvenate your brain – and start practising.

Don't stop dreaming

When Martin Luther King passionately told the American public that he had a dream, he tapped into a deep well of emotion in all human beings. Dreams are big, uplifting and grip the imagination. Having a dream is exciting and at the same time it's a call to action. Without a dream there is no motivation. And this is one thing in which Old Brains are singularly lacking.

Ask many an 80-year-old what their plans are for the future and you'll get a bizarre stare back. Plans! At my age! Are you pulling my leg? But why not?

It is frightening, moreover, to observe just how many 45-year-olds – or even 30-year-olds – lack a route map too. Somewhere along the line, dreams come to be seen to be for youngsters. Dreaming is not something a mature adult does.

Old Brains live much of their lives in the past tense. How they were when they were younger. How society was. And, oh! The great injustices that have befallen them in between times.

In Alain de Botton's *Essays in Love*, he defines this syndrome as 'psycho-fatalism', saying that some people [Old Brains] are 'bewildered and exhausted [they suffocate] on question marks: Why me? Why this? Why now?'

In this state of pessimism about life and everything around us, how is one to dream? How is one to get motivated? Rather, nightmares crowd in. As much as the past was better, the future is worse. So forget foresight. And forget having power over events or influencing the future.

With Old Brains, it often boils down to this realisation: 'Create the future? I can't even control the present.'

But whatever your age, 18 or 80, there are enormous paybacks to be gained from this Wisdom of Youth.

Read the following list and start imagining a better life for yourself.

Benefits of designing tomorrow

- Producing something special that gives pleasure to others (a drawing, garden or meal).
- Having an exciting dream; a vision for your unique life.
- Being fired up and enjoying the journey.
- Avoiding getting stale and predictable.
- Generating more efficient and effective ways of going about everyday life.
- Being recognised as an innovator and invited to join new ventures.
- Keeping family life fresh.
- Being confident in your ability to think your way out of difficult situations.
- Stimulating your interest in the creative works of others; enjoying the arts.
- Designing a home environment that gives you a thrill throughout the day.

- Marking your individuality (through dress, interests or creativity).
- Getting to the future first.
- Having something specific to hope for (recognised by psychologists as a key element in a happy life).

Adopt three 'designing tomorrow' mindsets as your own

Enjoying these benefits will require effort, as with all the wisdoms of youth.

The challenge is to review and accept the following three Young Brain mindsets which harness this wisdom:

1 Being Optimistic

2 Inventing Magic

3 Daring to Dream.

Smile and get reading:

1 Being optimistic

Optimism challenges

1 Do you believe that most things in life are impossible?

2 Is your initial reaction to new ideas usually 'It won't work' or 'It'll never catch on'?

Let's look on the bright side of life.

An historical truth

In terms of the evolution of the human race, it's pretty obvious that Young Brained optimists have been the key enablers of our development. They make more things happen than people who lack a positive outlook on life. Why bother to plant seeds in the spring if they probably won't come up in autumn? Why bother to fight off wolves or bears if they are bigger and stronger than you are? Or defend family or homeland, if the enemy will probably win anyway?

And optimism is no less relevant today – and a strong inner sense of purpose that goes naturally with a positive outlook.

The key issue is that optimists don't just hope for the best. Hope is a very positive thing but, without a plan and some action, it is weak and probably delusive. It is because optimists are committed and action-orientated, they get on with doing their level best to turn hope into reality.

Winston Churchill in 1939 was leading a nation that was facing almost impossible odds. Ill-prepared and alone, his country was seemingly at the mercy of the German air force at the outset of the Battle of Britain. He knew that some bloody-minded optimism was required. Once pessimism took over, it was a done deal and the Germans would win. Being a master psychologist himself, he was able to project the British public forward to a time when it could look back and say 'This was their finest hour.'

The evidence supporting the influence of optimists throughout history has been also validated by psychologists. They find that optimists do tend to be lopsided – they put a more rosy gloss on things than is justified by events – and believe themselves to have more control in certain situations than they actually do have. The upside is that they tend not be daunted by events, and as a result tend to achieve things against the odds.

There is also scientific evidence that optimists tend to live longer and have better health.

Living the Wisdom

The weight of scientific and historical evidence, plus common sense, makes being optimistic a no-brainer. A key to behaving as if the glass is half full is to nip negative and cynical thoughts in the bud. This requires great presence of mind and a real desire not to want to wallow in the mire of pessimism. Use that Young Brained 'self-talk' we mentioned earlier and always try to contradict any spontaneously negative reactions to events. Think of the glass as being half full – and mean it.

Pessimism is pernicious

'Start every day with a smile. Get it over with.'

W.C. Fields

It is important to understand how insidious the alternative to optimism is. Its opposite, pessimism, is potentially devastating for the human condition. It leads eventually to depression, largely because it induces a false sense of helplessness. Pessimists believe they cannot influence events, and their lack of positive action leads to a self-fulfilling prophecy.

Psychologists are clear that pessimists develop a sense of helplessness because they feel that nothing that they can do will affect the outcome of life around them. They become paralysed by their own sense of being swept along by negative happenings. Studies over the years have shown that pessimists achieve less, give up more easily and get depressed more readily. In the same studies, optimists tend to do better at school and college, work and in sport.

Living the Wisdom

Fight learned helplessness by taking 'the next step'. Any time you are set back and feel overwhelming pessimism, start designing a better tomorrow by making a small but positive step away from the problem. For example, if you've just heard that your house sale has fallen through, get decorating. The next 'buyer' needs to be so in love with your house that walking away from it would be unthinkable.

2 Inventing magic

Inventing magic challenges

1 Are you challenging yourself regularly to come up with exciting creative answers to improving things for the people around you?

2 Do you find complexity in the world worrying – or stimulating?

Okay. Ready to make some magic in your life?

An enchanting spell

Life is exhilarating for Young Brains for a simple reason. They work at making it so.

A predictable routine may be the reality, but it can be spiced up to be more unpredictable and exciting. The 9-to-5 existence besets even the Young Brain, but its instinctive wisdom tells it to make the most of this situation by creating unusual and rewarding events – at the very least on a daily basis.

They apply imagination to a dull, dreary existence and come up with inventive ideas to create happiness and daily enchantment.

In inventing magic, the Young Brain acknowledges that every living moment cannot be fun and rewarding, but life is for living and it's only worthwhile if interesting things are made to happen, and dreams are brought to fruition on a regular basis.

So, had a bad day at work? The old or Middle-aged Brain response is to go home and stew about it. The Young Brain says, how can I pick myself up, and get into a more positive and lively frame of mind? It seeks magic in a bar, a shopping mall, at the cinema, morphing into its avatar on *Second Life*, or even by dropping in unexpectedly on old friends in the real world. Although it might seem strange to the middle-aged or Old Brain, actively engaging with others, rather than moping by yourself in private, is all about making magic in your life.

More enchantment is to be had from the last-minute weekend break, or the visit to an elderly and much-loved relative.

---

lastminute.com, the company which sells off unsold tickets to events at the eleventh hour, has deservedly built its business fortune on seekers of magic. It provides tickets to events or destinations that either have not sold for their full asking price, or have been handed back because of unforeseen circumstances very late in the day. Its customers are often people seeking a lift to their spirits by a spontaneous decision to experience a concert or take in a show at short notice.

Tiny things, too, can create special moments. The small tattoo on the shoulder blade, some sexy new lingerie, a naughty but nice doughnut shared with a friend. Any excuse to do something very slightly unusual or illicit which provides a spurt of satisfaction or enjoyment. A daily buzz to liven up a dull day – it just requires a little touch of creativity to lift things from the mundane to the interesting or exciting.

A recent Viagra advertisement captured this perfectly. A middle-aged husband is seen tidying the kitchen and, opening a cupboard, happens upon lots of plastic containers. His eye catches the swimming pool in the yard and a glint appears. The viva viagra music plays as the voice-over suggests that it is important to keep life interesting. Cut to the husband and wife swimming in the twilight with the plastic lids floating majestically on the pool's surface supporting candles. A magic moment, holding the promise of still more interesting things to come.

While Pfizer, makers of Viagra, hold up the magical properties of their invention, it's evident that the real hero is the husband's imagination and his ability to cast enchanting spells.

The challenge, of course, facing Old Brains in this situation is that it is so easy to slip into cynicism. Had the man not been intent on trying to charm his wife, it is quite possible he would not have assembled and lit all the candles that were floating romantically on the pool. Male brains – especially middle-aged and Old Brains – tend to be a bit impatient with candles. They cost money, make a mess, and give an inadequate light to do anything by, especially eating!

So Old Brains – especially male Old Brains – need to resist the temptation towards cynicism, and rethink their attitudes to enchantment in all its forms. Romance and magic are easy to dismiss by short-tempered Old Brains as having no objective value or use. But, as Young Brains can confirm, they lead to interesting places.

Their use is that they help us move on from the pragmatic, functional day-to-day into the more imaginative and creative way of thinking that is natural to Young Brains. Their value is that they enable us to find the stardust to sprinkle on our day and life.

But inventing magic is also about creating a desirable environment for yourself at home. When you set the table to reflect the Thai food you are just about to serve your guests, you are inventing magic. When you light incense and put on Chopin or Jack Johnson while you're in the bath, you are creating a magical moment. When you put on a new deodorant or perfume to transform your mood, you are on a quest for olfactory enchantment. And even when you have Nirvana playing at 100 decibels, you seek an emotional rush.

It is so much easier for the mind to vegetate in front of the television and yet, with this kind of imaginative intelligence, your life can become so much more rewarding – every single day.

Creative Young Brains are looking to fulfil themselves in many areas of life as a direct result of their innovative outputs. However, it is noteworthy that the reward that is often most highly sought after is recognition.

It is recognition that gives glitter to any creative achievement. The reward lies in the recognition that their peer group gives to the creative work. In essence, Young Brains are seeking to be accepted as magicians.

Living the Wisdom

When you spring surprises and give gifts from the heart, everyone wins. So work at creating enchanting spells until it becomes an exhilarating, life-enhancing and necessary part of your life.

Benefiting from complexity

In their quest to invent magic, Young Brains cast their net far and wide. They draw on technology, multicultural influences and what they saw at the last craft fair. The joy of the Young

Brain is that it is adept at combining these sources and, in a process akin to alchemy, coming up with something new.

Combine touch screens and mobile phones and you get the iPhone, (Apple's Steve Jobs, of course, being a prime example of someone who is middle-aged but with a Young Brain). Add micro-encapsulation technology (a process used in scratch-and-sniff perfume samples you get inside magazines) to tattooing and you get revolutionary removable tattoos. Take people's desire to eat quality food and snack while on the move and you get gourmet fast food. The potential benefits of complexity are all around us and the Young Brain is enormously talented at putting one and one together to get three.

Or should it be putting one and one together to get thousands? The Young Brain has understood, with instinctive clarity, the power of the Internet community. Complexity is put to work to the benefit of everyone. Flickr is a website that shares contributors' photos with everyone else. From this apparent complexity, individuals can see and be stimulated by the creative work of the global village.

Similarly, the online encyclopaedia, Wikipedia, allows anyone with knowledge in a specialised area to capture it for the benefit of the global community. Everyone can contribute, edit and police – and everyone can benefit. These, and other instances of dynamic social networking, give new ways of benefiting from seeming complexity They add a huge chunk of value, and give Young Brains the raw materials needed to fuel their imaginations.

Older brains, on the other hand, tend to feel swamped by the richness of Web 2.0, and bemused by how complicated it all is. They tend to engage in reductionist thinking, rather than expansionist thinking. Facts, reason and analysis all conspire to make Old Brains shut off potential ways of imagining things or doing things in new ways. The 'not invented here' syndrome is a classic example of reductionist thinking.

Benefiting from complexity defines the Young Brain's expansionist capacity to see only opportunity in the cornucopia of modern life.

Living the Wisdom

Determine to embrace the excitement, richness and potential of complexity, and relish the fresh insights and cross-fertilisation it can stimulate. Got a presentation to make at work? Draw on parallels from unrelated industries to bring new insights. Building a shed in the garden? Why not be inspired by pagodas and make life a little more quirky?

---

3 Daring to dream

Dream challenges

1 Do you have a creative project that you are incubating or realising at the moment?

2 Do you enjoy exploring imaginary/virtual worlds (science fiction works, video games, fantasy gaming, surreal art, historical novels, etc.)?

Time to step into dreamland . . .

Regressing to childhood

The Young Brain has the capacity to summon up the child within and, in so doing, live each day with creativity and imagination. Adulthood has many things to commend it, but it does little to sustain imaginations. Think back, for a moment, to your own childhood. Maybe you had imaginary friends, or a fantasy world for your dolls or Action Men. You almost certainly role-played doctors and nurses, and cowboys and Indians with friends.

Living inside your head came naturally and you often startled unsuspecting adults as you sought to incorporate them into your own fantasy. Well then, what happened? That's a big question but the short answer is that education – particularly school education – happened.

'Throughout our lives we are trained to do the right thing, the right way. It begins with our parents, continues in school and gets reinforced at work … by doing so we often lose the ability … to think tangentially and solve our puzzles in a creative way.'

Chris Barez-Brown, *How to Have Kick-ass Ideas*, 2006

So, the Young Brain has figured out that to be creative or inventive, it has to revert to childhood – in the jargon, it has to undertake regression.

The Young Brain puts itself into a childlike state by joking, letting go of appearances, refusing to be embarrassed or trying things out. Most importantly, it experiments through play.

In business, companies such as Ford, Visteon, JWT, Orange (to name but a very few) have rooms full of Lego, Fuzzy Felt, Rubik's cubes and other tactile puzzles, to encourage staff to regress to their more creative infancy. *What If* is a very successful worldwide innovation agency. Its innovation process starts with 'helping people to discover their own personal creative genius' and its advice for getting creative movement and momentum: 'find life funny'. According to *What If*, the recipe for staying exactly where you are – in other words, to be an Old Brain – is: 'To be serious! To take it seriously! Take yourself seriously'

(Chris Barez-Brown, *How to Have Kick-ass Ideas*, 2006).

Advertising and design agencies have long since come to the same conclusion. From table tennis and pool tables in head office basements to hosting weekday parties, creativity is fuelled by regressive activities.

The best teachers realise this too. They are still in daily contact with the child within. They're good at their jobs because they can continually adapt and relate to their students. Not by superficially wearing the same clothes as them, or adopting the same figures of speech, but by being contemporary in their values and attitudes.

They don't compromise their principles, which are timeless, but they do – because they are always involved with young people – instinctively update their attitudes and values so that they fit seamlessly into the youthful context. They still have the same wonder, excitement and imagination of the children they teach. They are childlike, yet have the authority of adults.

There are other professions, too, where regression is important for success.

'[Theatre is] the happiest haven for those who have secretly put their childhood in their pockets, so they continue to play to the end of their days.'

Max Reinhardt, 1928, founder of the Salzburg Festival

Daring to dream – pre-imagining a desirable outcome – is powerful whatever age you are and whatever change you want to happen. Dreams come in all shapes, sizes, colours and flavours. A dream can be the creation of a better relationship with a difficult relative, or having a more abundant social life, or just getting better at an activity you enjoy taking part in. Whatever it is, once you can imagine it, the creative juices in your mind get to work to find positive ways to make it happen.

As a result, there is a very strong likelihood it will happen, however unlikely it may look now.

Young Brains instinctively know this, as we stated earlier, and consequently tend to attribute greater importance to having a dream than do older brains. They also attach more importance to the kind of dreams you dream when you are asleep. For an Old Brain, such a dream may be satisfying but lead to nothing in particular. For a Young Brain, they are a jumping-off point. Stephen King, the hugely successful author of horror stories, claims to get many of his best ideas from his dreams. Many influential songwriters say they wake with a tune in their heads. Many inventors keep a notebook by their bed for when a great idea strikes them in the midnight hour. In all cases, the belief is that dreams are significant, contain important, often original information, and need to be recognised for their worth.

Picasso's quotation at the beginning of this book is profoundly true: 'Every child is born an artist. The trick is to remain an artist.' Creativity has a childlike openness and optimism about it – a belief that anything is possible, anything can be created. It also requires the will to stick at it – like a child endlessly playing the same games, wanting to read the same stories – and finding something fresh in them each time.

Living the Wisdom

Put a notebook and pencil on your bedside table and be prepared to jot down your dreams when you stir in the night. Take time, the following day, to ask: 'What is this dream telling me/showing me?' Above all, be prepared to be inspired to creativity through your dreams.

Part of the new elite

Today, dreaming is not for dreamers. Far from being *Billy Liar* types, dreamers are now productive and respected members of society. Suddenly, the creative professions are highly valued.

It used to be that, if you were artistic, you were seen by society at large to be rather flaky, somewhat lazy and certain of a life of suffering for your art. Artists were mostly poor and were as unpredictable as their incomes. And everyone knows that even some famous artists died poor and lonely – Mozart and Van Gogh to name but two.

How things have changed. Creative people have now assumed an almost mystical status in our society. We have artists in abundance, and they touch our hearts and our souls with their music, dance, theatre and art. They make us cry, make us angry, make us ... human. And we are very willing to pay a king's ransom for such a valuable service. Madonna is one of the world's richest women. Artists such as Damien Hirst are feted wherever they go. Actors such as Tom Cruise and Eva Longoria have the world at their feet. Not to mention J.K. Rowling, the fabulously wealthy creator of *Harry Potter*.

And ask yourself. Are the people we have just mentioned Old Brains or Young Brains? Yes, the creative spark of the new elite arises from Young Brain thinking.

And attaining wealth through creativity is increasingly democratic. You only have to look at American urban rappers to see the truth of this. Across much of America, if you are poor you have three paths to obtain wealth – sport, crime or music. The term 'gangsta rap' suggests that many try more than one pathway.

For those who succeed on the creative track like 50 Cent and Eminem – fame and fortune await. Hip-hop represents a way to breakout, and in thousands of basements and garages across

America (and the world), Young Brains are using their creative talents to try to produce the next global soundtrack.

Meanwhile, it's not just creative Young Brains in the arts world who are grabbing the headlines. The world seemed to stop every time Apple's Steve Jobs ran his famous press conferences. What had his genius Californian engineers come up with? And what was next?

> In a ritual towards the end of his keynotes, Steve Jobs would feign to leave the stage then turn and say 'and one more thing ….' In the past this 'bonus' has heralded the PowerBook, iPod, MacBook Pro, iTunes store, Safari and iPhone.

Meanwhile, 'the new age of creativity' is acknowledged as being one of the ten forces that have been responsible for creating our globalised twenty-first century 'flat World', according to analyst Thomas L. Friendman.

In fact, daring to dream has become so far engrained in our culture that a whole generation has been defined in this way. Trendspotting.com has called this the C Generation, while Paul Ray and Sherry Ruth Anderson coined the term 'cultural creatives' and found 50 million Americans who hold creative world views, values and lifestyles. We simply call them Young Brains.

Living the Wisdom

If, like many people, you are bemused by a lot of the creative arts, focus your attention on just one school or even one artist that you take an instant fancy to. Learn about the art itself, the historical context and its influences. Once you feel comfortable, spread out your knowledge and passion to a neighbouring 'wave'. Your objective is not to be a know-all but to feel the emotion and to understand a little bit more about why the artist makes you feel that way.

Better by design

Good design leaves most Old Brains stone cold.

Unsurprisingly, Young Brains are in the vanguard of society's rising appreciation of design. Daring to dream is also about daring to want to have beautiful things in our lives. In our public buildings, our private dwellings, our clothes and the products we buy and use. We are now more design aware than ever before, and none more so than Young Brains.

Whether it's the Guggenheim Museum in Bilbao, Spain, the Milhau Bridge floating through the clouds 300 metres from the ground in central France, the Sydney Opera House, the Walt Disney Concert Hall in Los Angeles, or Taipei 101, people are passionate about brave and imaginative buildings, and travel great distances just to see them. The very fact they are now called 'iconic' demonstrates their importance in our sensibilities.

Inside art galleries, the exhibits aren't just more popular, their presentation is getting more imaginative and diverse. Curators around the world have gained new energy and encouragement. Tate Modern in London, for example, even allowed its massive brick façade to be used for giant graffiti, to publicise an exhibition on the subject – unimaginable just a few years ago.

Meanwhile, the art and fashion communities come ever closer together. Expect to see more examples of art-inspired fashion over the next few years as well as art exhibitions in your favourite clothing store.

Donald Trump is a great example of a Young Brain in an old body. Here's what one of the world richest men has to say about aesthetics: 'Everyone knows how important beauty is to me. I always try to have it in my life. Being surrounded by beauty makes me feel great; it enhances every part of my life, and I deserve it. For me, style and success are completely inter-woven. I wouldn't want to have one without the other. When you have beauty in your life, it can make everything better and more worthwhile.'

Donald Trump, *Trump 101*

Young Brains have a hunger for style. For them the continual pursuit of good design means choosing a digital camera because of the look and feel; choosing an Apple Mac over a PC due to its funkier user interface and 'lickable' surface design – even picking a brand of peas because the label has a more stylish impact. As the world takes on a new designer look, Young Brains know that a heightened ability to discern the inherent aesthetic appeal of things is one key to creating a more pleasing and satisfying life.

Simply put, design satisfies the basic human desire for beauty. Young Brains embrace it, because it inspires them and gives them joy. You too can share in this joy.

Living the Wisdom

Find ways to enjoy good design. A simple technique is to promote good design up your list of reasons why you choose to buy a certain item. If your toaster has broken down, you may end up paying more for a good-looking new one, but you can always compensate by skipping something non-essential for a few weeks. The gain is that you'll enjoy that strikingly beautiful object in your kitchen for many years to come.

SUMMARY OF GOALS

Being able to stimulate and open up your imagination and creativity is one of the great blessings of having a Young Brain. Optimism is a natural precursor of happiness and fulfillment, and both are enhanced by daily enchantment, and dreaming of the future.

- Be positive about the future – believe you can make it yours.
- Do something different and special every day – make magic.
- Dream big.

09

Why successful groups need Young Brains

We have spent most of this book describing how individuals can boost their YQs by adopting the six wisdoms of youth. We've referred to families, associations, businesses, institutions and so on but it's always been from the perspective of how one person can change his or her life. Only by inference have we vaguely perceived how the social groups themselves might benefit.

However, we are confident that, as you have read this book, it has been obvious that Young Brain thinking can be of enormous benefit to groups of people and even to society at large.

Imagine how dynamic a community, a region or even a nation would be if the majority of its people – of whatever chronological age – were Young Brained? Would we even have to talk so much about an ageing population if many more people demonstrated the virtues of youthfulness? And wouldn't companies be more successful if fed by the flexibility, energy and creativity of Young Brain thinking?

Let's, briefly, look at several different groups in turn and point out how much more successful they would be with Young Brains at the helm and on the deck.

Young Brained families

'Few parents nowadays pay any regard to what their children say to them. The old-fashioned respect for the young is fast dying out.'

Oscar Wilde

Are families dysfunctional by definition? Absolutely not – but very few reach the heights of perfect harmony either! Having more Young Brains inside the family unit would certainly help since many arguments start – and continue – because of Old

Brain attitudes and actions. The following are some of the ways that Old Brains plunge families into disharmony:

- They refuse to travel – relatives have to come to visit them.
- They are always out of sorts and reserve a poor welcome to those who love them most.
- Not wanting to change, they create physical discomfort for those around them: their heating doesn't work well; they sit in the only comfortable chair; their car lets in water.
- They need people to agree with them, provoking frustration in others and a lack of resolution on important issues.
- They make high demands on the family's time, since a lack of close friends means they are too dependent on their relations.
- They tend to get sick more than the average; as the phrase goes, they are 'high maintenance'.
- A lack of laughter means that tensions can never be tackled by a simple joke diffuse to the situation.

Clearly, this list is far from exhaustive but perhaps you recognised some issues as being bugbears in your family. Too close for comfort? Well, then use this book to rejuvenate yourself and give copies to those family members who need to adopt a younger spirit. With several relations on the same rejuvenation agenda, you might find the whole unit benefits from things such as:

- closer contact and cooperation
- a new spirit of generosity
- more laughter and renewed interest in spending time together
- a willingness to talk about tensions and get them off the table
- more intergenerational understanding and less criticism of the younger children

- more empathy with young parents and their approach to bringing up their children
- the use of modern communications technology to be more involved and relevant in each others' lives
- fewer couch potatoes; a more lively atmosphere where new activities together become possible
- a more fair-minded and context-specific sharing of roles and tasks between the male and female family members.

Again, not an exhaustive list, but surely even these changes would go a long way to improving everyone's satisfaction within the family.

Young Brained associations and clubs

One of the biggest struggles for most societies is membership. Dwindling numbers are putting the very existence of the group at risk. Sound familiar? Well, one huge benefit of attracting Young Brains to join is that they are well connected. Not only do they easily fit in with existing members but, if they find what they are looking for, they will start to invite their extended network too. Membership can really snowball and suddenly you have all the resources you need to be a successful, vibrant organisation.

But how to attract them in the first place? Here, honesty is the best course of action. Is your club a Young Brained club? Is it flexible, action-oriented, adventurous, light-hearted, creative, open minded and so on. If not, chances are you've not got many Young Brains on board at present – so how can you hope to introduce new youthful members in the future?

The first action associations should aim for is to rejuvenate what they currently do, with the current membership. Once again, if key members had access to the tools and approaches outlined in this book, and began to rejuvenate, an unstoppable momentum could be created. And once the association is past its Young Brained 'tipping point', attracting dynamic, youthful members from outside becomes not only possible but probable.

Success will come when:

- change becomes natural and desirable
- new members are accepted with open arms – fresh blood is always welcome
- meetings are one of the highlights of everyone's week – always informative and fun
- asking for volunteers becomes easy; everyone wants to be involved somewhere
- prizes are valued, not disdained. People want recognition from peers they respect
- money flows in; new joins and new generosity fill the coffers and keeps the treasurer busy
- excursions are full to the brim; everyone wants to go
- the organisation becomes less hierarchical; people do things because they want to not because someone tells them to.

Young Brained companies

Successful companies are businesses that understand, implicitly, the society in which they operate and can then tune in to its many demands and opportunities.

By understanding Young Brains (and how they differ from older brains), businesses and institutions pinpoint much of what they need to know about what is going on in society at large and can start to anticipate how this might change in the future.

Successful companies will want to attract Young Brained customers with Young Brained products and services. They will also need to recruit and retain higher numbers of Young Brained staff – while, of course, retraining older brains by helping them to rejuvenate. Finally, to be successful will increasingly require a company to run Young Brain business processes. Let's look at these briefly one at a time. (For more information, click on author Chris Middleton's website at: www.futurescoaching.com)

Young Brained customers

At one level, all companies need to research Young Brains since they access change so easily and are so much part of the future. Being successful means analysing and understanding the motivations of these cutting-edge segments, even if they are not customers.

For many companies, however, Young Brains will be part of the customer base who 'walk through their doors' every day of the week.

At this level, marketers would do well to have an answer to the question: What proportion of my current customer base have Young Brains and what am I doing to appeal directly to their needs? A second key question for marketers to understand is: Is it desirable that the Young Brained segment becomes my main target customer? It is certainly true that Young Brains should be attractive to many industries – including technology, cosmetics, electronic goods and leisure sectors.

Another question begging a response is: How will Young Brains be different tomorrow? In other words, what are the trends that continue to shape the youthful mindset?

Answers to these and other targeting, positioning and branding questions need careful analysis and knowledgeable responses. But the first step is to find and talk to Young Brains.

Young Brain products and services

Today, many companies make the mistake of assuming that only teenagers and young adults are youthful. But, as we have seen, you can have a Young Brain at any age. From this error comes the idea that youthful products and services need to be designed with only teenagers and young adults in mind. And so we get lots of focus on street culture and fashions and fads – often American in origin. These products are possibly cheaper too – in order to fit pocket money and first salary purchase potential.

But a successful Young Brained company will realise that many Young Brains are older, sometimes richer and more often have children than the popular misconception.

So what about inventing the video game for the Young Brained family man? Or the intuitive (rather than complex) luxury car? How about pension products that are fun? Or trains with 'networking' carriages specifically for people who are open to others and who want to spend the journey talking to anyone and everyone?

The Young Brain phenomenon is a rich, deep source of innovation and successful companies will be the ones to tap into this seam.

Young Brained employees

Young Brains are essential in any company or institution. Why they are super-attractive to employers? Here is a list:

- They are up with the trends.
- They don't resist, rather they welcome change.
- They are informed workers and communicate naturally.
- They are always on, ready for action.

- They work well in teams; for example, they are less likely to be sexist, racist, etc.

- They are savvy and take quick, intuitive decisions.

- They are not tied to tradition, so work well as innovators.

- They are upbeat and energetic, no matter what their age.

- They are technological natives.

- They are fun to be with.

- They are always learning and developing.

- They welcome mobility and expanding their horizons.

- They are lucky.

Sound like a dream team? You bet! A first step in the right direction for any HR manager would be to deploy our fuller Brain Age Test to measure staff YQs, followed by team assessments and coaching older brains to rejuvenate. Wouldn't you want your company run by Young Brains?

On a more depressing note, successful companies are also the ones that weed out older-brained elements. This fear of being left on the shelf should be enough to drive any sensible employee to think themselves younger.

Young Brain processes

It's not enough, of course, to have Young Brain employees, if they are not productive. In the future, successful companies will be the ones that revitalise their very business processes to make the most of all their youthful talent.

For example, how many businesses run innovation processes that flop because they are not Young Brained enough? The brainstorming process can be predicable, uninspiring and not oriented to the future. Ironic, isn't it? And yet there are dynamic approaches to innovation that get the Young Brain juices really flowing. Success in innovation means knowing how.

Companies who've 'got it'

What are some of the Young Brained companies out there? Clearly tech companies such as Apple, Google, The Geek Squad and Orange are Young Brained and so too are many (but not all) creative, ad and design agencies. Lynx is a racy Young Brained toiletries brand – but so too is the more down-to-earth Dove. Toyota and Harley Davidson are young at heart, while in clothing, Diesel, Nike and Oakley are among those that just keep moving forward. The list goes on . . . Absolut Vodka, Virgin Atlantic, Innocent Smoothies and many more – you get the point.

And the one thing that unifies these companies is that Young Brains actively want to work for them. They become self-perpetuating. A Young Brained company attracts Young Brained employees who energise and rejuvenate the company once more. Talk about a virtuous circle.

Meanwhile, just try attracting Young Brains to an Old Brained company. They are too slow, unadventurous, local and TOO SERIOUS! Anecdotes are rife of Young Brains being asked in to be interviewed, only to be told that they will not be given their own laptop – at least not immediately – and simply walking out of the interview. Companies are either 'with it' or 'against it'.

Other winning groups

What about other social groups? Would they also benefit from having Young Brains on board? You had better believe it. Charities would raise more funds if they recruited volunteers who were more proactive and enlightened. And their fundraisers would arguably be of a more solid profile if they had achieved a good balance between selflessly helping others and attending to their own sense of self-worth.

Public institutions, too, might be able to rejuvenate their mandate and mission with an infusion of Young Brained talent. Today, our public service is dominated by conservative forces which actually hold them back from servicing the public's changing needs. More Young Brain staff and processes would place public institutions on the highway to the future.

For example, in education it would be good to see students being taught the virtues of Adaptive Navigation rather than being led to believe that there is normally a reliable route between A and B. Life is more complex and variable than our education system implies, and arming students with this insight would send them into the world with more realistic assumptions.

Finally, of course, society at large would benefit from raising its YQ. Being more adapted to the realities of modern living, a Young Brained society will perform better economically, be more at ease with itself socially and, combining both, be healthier and happier. Social rejuvenation. What could be wiser than that?

10

Eternal Youth

We've covered quite a bit of ground over the last nine chapters. In the process we have handed you two very powerful things. Firstly, we have revealed the Wisdom of Youth. It is the wisdom to erase fear and do what young people do when they know nothing. It is natural and extremely effective in modern society.

But we hope that we've also given you new ambition. The ambition to believe in yourself, the desire to make the most of opportunities that life presents and the conviction that it is absolutely possible to remake and renew your life.

In fact, this whole book has been about the opportunity to change yourself. By changing your mindset and adopting the Wisdom of Youth you can become more open, flexible, energetic, courageous, joyful, enthusiastic, optimistic, creative, fulfilled and effective. Rediscovering the Wisdom of Youth truly does liberate you to be young again.

Where does your ambition stop?

Is this enough for you? If this book achieves everything we mention above will you be satisfied? You will be younger, more relevant and more self-assured. Is that enough?

What about eternal youth?

Clearly we have no magic elixir allowing you to live physically for ever. But the nearest thing to eternal youth we know of is leaving a legacy. In other words, to be remembered long after you are dead – for your memory to be eternal.

This is a step change in ambition level. Rather than just leading a full and youthful life, you do so in a way that benefits posterity. Surely this is the definition of *real* success in life.

For most of us, leading a good life – and avoiding the traps of Old Brainhood – is enough. However, if you do aspire to eternal youth, how should you go about it? This is what we address in this chapter.

Achieving eternal youth

Who has achieved eternal youth? Well, remembering your history classes already gives you a first idea. Famous leaders, scientists, discoverers, artists, philanthropists – all by virtue of their contribution to society – are remembered down the ages.

But eternal youth can be achieved at a very local scale too. Benefactors who bequeath buildings and local worthies who support the less advantaged also live long in the memory.

At yet another scale, within individual families, many people get forgotten, but one or two become legends due to their unique contribution, and they survive across the generations.

So, you don't necessarily have to make a breakthrough technological discovery or give millions to local charity to be remembered. Being a hero to your own family and friends can get you a long way into the future.

Going beyond the Wisdom of Youth: The Wisdom of Experience

For all the reasons we have explained, regaining the Wisdom of Youth is essential if you want to remain relevant and happy in your lifetime. However, if you want eternal youth, it is still not enough. If you want to be remembered long after your death, you have to combine youthful wisdom with another kind of wisdom. This is the Wisdom of Experience which we referred to in Chapter 1.

The Wisdom of Experience is something we learn over time. As we live, we learn hard lessons about life. And the longer we live, hopefully, the more lessons we learn. This is what we mean when we talk about the Wisdom of Experience.

It is, then, the result of good judgement and insights remembered. It balances means and ends judiciously. And the people exhibiting it tend to exhibit also the trait of human kindness. And they understand that clear standards and boundaries, plus encouragement, always ultimately work better than arbitrary laws and coercion.

Of course, not everyone learns the Wisdom of Experience well. Many people go through life making the same mistakes time and again. But the wise try to make sense of problems and tragedies; and they attempt to see rules and reason behind luck and opportunities.

There is a fuller story to be told about the wisdom of experience but our purpose is not to tell it here. However, for those whose ambition stretches to eternal youth, a very abbreviated analysis follows.

Like the Wisdom of Youth, the Wisdom of Experience is made up of six elements:

1 A Strong Moral Compass

2 The Importance of Roots

3 The Importance of Others

4 Tomorrow Exists as well as Today

5 The Realities of Life

6 An Enviable Equanimity

1 A Strong Moral Compass

As we get more experience of human behaviour we come to have a pretty deep understanding of the difference between right and wrong. Life has opened our eyes to the problems and stresses that arise if we ignore our conscience when we are in a difficult situation.

Chickens are relentless in the way they come home to roost. We learn not to fudge issues on what are, usually, simple issues of morality. We learn to try to do the right thing, however uncomfortable, because if we don't we know it will come back and bite us.

Experience also teaches that politeness is not old-fashioned and irrelevant. It costs nothing and lubricates social transactions. We learn over time that there is a whole world of difference between sexual openness and promiscuity. Moreover, we come to understand that personal freedom has to be counterbalanced with personal responsibility.

2 The Importance of Roots

When we are young, where we come from is vaguely interesting but not very important. Our sights are firmly set on the future. The past is tied up with strange cousins, aunts and uncles, some of whom give credence to the old saying that friends are God's apology for relations.

As we get older, especially if we have children ourselves, we become intensely aware of the love that can bind families, and the significant influence both individuals and places in our family's past can play in our evolution as fully formed personalities. We become more interested in our family history and our origins in order to better understand our own family context and our role within that context.

3 The Importance of Others

This is a widening out of the importance of roots. In our youth we tend to be obsessed with ourselves. Indeed, at times in adolescence, we exist in a kind of subjective idealism in which other people are merely projections of our imaginations.

Life appears to revolve around us, and we are self-centred to a degree that is, on reflection, embarrassing. How different this form of introspective selfishness is from enlightened selfishness. Rather than centring all our attention on ourselves and what benefits *us*, we are, in our enlightenment, creating space for ourselves to grow as individuals, so we can give back *more* to other people – our family, our friends or our community.

This is because, as the years pass, we come to realise that other people don't just exist, they are central to our existence and our happiness. Our self-esteem, our fulfilment, our effectiveness as human beings are all anchored in our capacity to acknowledge the importance of other human beings.

This is sometimes a difficult lesson to learn, but it is part of the personal growth that needs to take place in the passage to maturity.

4 Tomorrow exists as well as Today

Comprehending that actions – and sometimes, more importantly, the absence of actions – have consequences, is something that youth can be slow to learn. Working, or not working hard for exams, applying oneself, or not applying oneself to a job, are often decisions taken with reference to peer group pressure, or personal convenience or whim, rather than with a view to their impact on future employability or income.

The confidence that the future will take care of itself is one of the things that make youth so attractive. *Carpe diem* – harvesting the day – comes naturally to the young. But it can be in a kind of vacuum, because the fruits of the harvest are consumed as they are harvested.

As we gain experience of life, we harvest the day but retain some of the fruits, because we know we need to have the seeds to plant for tomorrow's harvest.

Making decisions that impact on the future, and understanding their impacts, is what separates man from the animals. Increasing maturity increases our understanding of this and makes us better at it.

5 The Realities of Life

Naivety and youth are natural bedfellows. When young, we understand some of the realities of life, but experience of them brings an emotional – and therefore deeper – understanding too.

It is a waste of breath to tell a young person that he or she is naive. We wouldn't have believed it when we were young, so why should we expect them to believe it now? Contrary to the belief of many young people, bills, overdrafts and credit cards eventually have to be repaid, and if they're your debts, then you have to pay them.

Maturity brings a deep insight into how life works. It's seldom fair, it's often challenging, and there are no free lunches. We may not relish it. But at least we know how it works, and can get some satisfaction out of making a good fist of it.

6 An Enviable Equanimity

Equanimity sounds pretty dull, but it's a whole lot better than stress and anxiety. There is a saying that you should always be thankful for bad luck – it's the only kind of luck you're going to get. It's not true, of course, but sometimes it may feel that way.

Raging against the world and its injustices transmutes in maturity into a sense that the best way to deal with the slings and arrows of outrageous fortune is to grin and bear it. The grin part is important. It's not just the ability to cope with life's upsets, it's the development of an unflappable maturity that allows us to sustain them with equanimity and good humour.

The growing capacity to behave with grace under pressure is one of the greatest boons of increasing years.

Staying younger and feeling sharper

Your best chance of eternal youth is to mesh the Wisdom of Youth and the wisdom of experience into a very powerful combination. By doing so, you will begin to lead a revitalised life.

Wisdom of Youth + Wisdom of experience = Revitalised Life

It is worth confirming that fusing the Wisdom of Youth and the Wisdom of Experience transcends the Young Brain/Old Brain distinction we've been referring to. You will increase your possibilities to obtain eternal youth if and when you start living a Revitalised life.

Benefits of mixing the Wisdom of Youth with the wisdom of experience

Recognising the strengths of the wisdom of experience allows you to moderate some of the excesses of the Wisdom of Youth:

- You can stay out late – but you don't feel that you have to.
- You could sleep on a friend's sofa – but only if you wanted to.
- You can participate on the charity committee – but not to the exclusion of your adult education course.
- You can change your values – but only to those that are morally justifiable.

Equally, having the Wisdom of Youth firmly in mind enables you to temper the excesses of wisdom of experience:

- Tomorrow is important – but you are also allowed to have fun today.
- Equanimity prevents ulcers – but excitement keeps you interested in life.

In other words, by fusing both wisdoms, you get the best of both worlds. Aiming for eternal youth is wise – and fun!

However, combining the two wisdoms is not just about one wisdom toning down the other. The fact is that they fuse into a pretty powerful set of benefits. Here are a few of them:

- Your can have a dream that excites you and others (designing tomorrow) and also know that it is an honourable and worthy one (strong moral compass).
- Your new energy and enthusiasm for life will supercharge your efforts to make a difference (being always on), and part of that difference will be to your family and those close to you (importance of roots).
- Your expanded sociability and liking for others (fresh blood) will

make you an uplifting presence, and more effective at rebuilding relationships with family members which may have decayed or become problematical (importance of roots).

- Your new optimism and positive approach – and the fact you're fun to be with – will make you a magnet to others (designing tomorrow/hedonistic high) and keep your relationships in good repair (importance of others).

- The self-confidence and people skills you have developed (enlightened selfishness) will enable you to lead and work with others more collaboratively and effectively (understanding that tomorrow exists as well as today).

- You are now more open to fresh ideas and, indeed, are the source of innovation (designing tomorrow) which makes you a powerhouse in improving the future (tomorrow exists as well as today).

- Your new courage to fight your corner (being always on and enlightened selfishness) will help you see things through to a positive conclusion however tough things get (the realities of life).

- Your evolving ability to manage your time intelligently (being always on) means you can balance high pace with savouring time, or being in the flow, which takes away stress and increases happiness (enviable equanimity).

SUMMING UP

The good news about accepting the challenge of increasing your YQ by adopting the Wisdom of Youth, and then combining it with the wisdom of experience, is that it is in your hands. You can self-medicate. There is no need to purchase expensive treatments, undergo risky cosmetic operations or take wonder drugs. There are no expensive makeover experts to pay. The only makeover is by you, *of you*.

At this time, we recommend that you to revisit the various chapters of the book where you either can see the quickest benefits – or the greatest need – and start to invest effort to make changes to your values, your comfort zones and your daily behaviours.

As you review your stepping-off point, remember that too many of us practise only what we are already good at; we neglect the skills that need more work. Why? Simply put, because it is frustrating to face up to repeated failure. It's much more satisfying to practise what you excel in. Avoid this temptation and give yourself the best possible chance to become young again. It's in your hands.

If you find it challenging at first, as we've said repeatedly, don't despair. We understand how significant a challenge this might be. After all, we are asking you not only to rethink some of your values, but also to change some behaviours which may be engrained and therefore rather uncomfortable to leave behind. But to have reached the end of the book shows that you want to take responsibility for your life – you are not a victim. And while it may take a lot of practice and reinforcement to incorporate new concepts into your behaviour, it is overwhelmingly worth the effort. Review the 'benefits' section of each wisdom to remind yourself why. You can – and *will* – succeed in increasing your Youth Quotient, and along with it your love of life.

Let us say it once again. If your aim is to be more youthful, you simply have to take actions along the lines detailed in this book. We have helped you identify the problem, shown you some practical actions to take and, hopefully, given you new ambition. However, there is a huge difference between knowing what the problem is and solving it. Put another way, this is the gap between having wisdom and living a Revitalised Life. We have put a very powerful set of wisdoms in your hands. Now it's up to you whether you use them; it's your choice to live a wise, and young, life.

At the beginning of the book you took the Brain Age Test to establish a snapshot of where your Youth Quotient was then. We suggest you go back to Chapter 2 now and take it again to benchmark your progress.

It is unlikely that you have become Young Brained overnight. If you have, congratulations, but try taking it again in a few weeks time to make sure your score wasn't influenced by over-excitement or a desire to give the answers your new understanding makes you feel more appropriate.

Do be scrupulously honest. The questions are the same as last time, so you can measure your progress over time. Which means the multiple responses will be the same. This is not a memory test – just answer spontaneously and genuinely.

Is your YQ increasing?

First, update the record you made in Chapter 2

My birthdays:

YQ now

Date:

My brain age (old, middle-aged or young):

Now, be ambitious and set yourself a **new** challenge:

My YQ Goal:

The strong likelihood is that there is quite a bit more work to do to reach your youthful ambitions. However, if you have already seen a measurable change to your YQ, pat yourself on the back.

We'd love to hear about your success. Email us with your story at: chris@futurescoaching.com

Top ten values

It may be too soon to retest your top values, because values change more slowly than attitudes. But if you cast your mind back to the example in Chapter 3 where we suggested that values such as fun, openness, enthusiasm and responsiveness might start to creep up your list in terms of importance. Do these already look more attractive and appropriate?

Look again at your top ten values in a few months time to see what has changed. Use the long list in Chapter 3 as a basis, and see what values you now find extremely important. And which you find less so.

The future

So it's over to you. We hope you've enjoyed reading the book as much as we have enjoyed writing it. We hope, also, we've given you some insights and tools that can quite literally change your life.

If you can invest the time and effort to work your way back to being Young Brained, it will make your life a whole lot more fun. And, combining that with the wisdom of experience, probably a whole lot more worthwhile too.

All you have to do is to be ready to ditch your Old Brain. For your Old Brain really is the elephant in the room. Everyone avoids talking about it, and tries to ignore it – including yourself. It's a huge presence, and one that can trample on your life chances.

So liberate yourself from dysfunctional thinking, and reject your Old Brain. Because **you can be as young as you think**!

Go for it – and good luck.